# ONE STEP AT A TIME

A royalty from every book sold is being given to the
Northwick Park Arthritis and Rheumatism Club

MARIE JOSEPH

# One Step at a Time

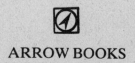

ARROW BOOKS

Arrow Books Limited
17–21 Conway Street, London W1P 6JD

An imprint of the Hutchinson Publishing Group

London Melbourne Sydney Auckland
Johannesburg and agencies
throughout the world

First published by Heinemann 1976
Arrow edition 1982

Set in Linoterm Times by
Book Economy Services
Burgess Hill, Sussex

Made and printed in Great Britain by
The Anchor Press Ltd
Tiptree, Essex

ISBN 0 09 928810 9

# FOR FRANK

Although the characters and situations in the book are real, the doctors and patients at the specialist hospital described have been given pseudonyms, and are not recognizable.　　　　M. J.

# FOREWORD

The foreword to the original edition of this book was written by my predecessor at Mount Vernon Hospital, Dr Francis Bach. Besides his merits as a physician, he was an exceptionally kind person, interested in his patients as well as in their illnesses. If all patients were like Marie Joseph, the practice of medicine might be very different. Her lively mind shines out throughout her book, with her ability to find out more about her illness and to assess in her own mind what her doctors have told her and to balance it with what she has learnt for herself. Until I read her book for the first time, and I have read it many times, I had little idea from her that she knew so much about the disease for which I treat so many people, and never was I given the idea that much of what I told her was not new to her. Perhaps I learnt more about the importance of a close relationship between doctor and patient from this book, and in particular how strongly the personalities of the people who treated her came over and may have been crucial factors in determining how she responded to her treatment. I recognized many of the doctors who had treated her and was surprised that she knew so much about so many of them – not obvious features – but of their character. I had greater difficulty in recognizing some of the patients she met in my ward, and only yesterday identified the James Bond girl.

Marie Joseph's account of her experience with rheumatoid arthritis now spans three and a half decades.

Those years have seen great changes in the practice of medicine, and enormous strides in the scientific understanding and treatment of disease. In the 1940s physicians were more concerned in the desperate fight to save lives of healthy young people taken suddenly and desperately ill with pneumonia or other infections and orthopaedic surgeons in treating the aftermath of poliomyelitis, tuberculous arthritis and osteomyelitis. Those physicians interested in rheumatic diseases were involved with rheumatic fever, a desperately serious disease, with wards full of people in the aftermath of rheumatic fever, which is the innocent involvement and partial destruction of the heart by the human body's natural response to deal with the streptococcal infection that caused the rheumatic fever. In this way we started to learn about autoimmunity, in which the body starts to attack different parts of itself with its own defence mechanisms. In some, rheumatic fever for instance, we have learnt about immunological recognition markers that heart muscle shares with streptococcal antigens, and which our body's immune system is incapable of distinguishing. In others we still have little other than a firmly held conviction that some unknown virus infection must change some of our genetic material held in every cell of the body so that it either becomes programmed to attack parts of the body or that it is no longer recognised as self by the defence mechanisms. Rheumatoid arthritis is one of the latter type of disease. One of the first major rheumatic disease centres was opened in the late 1930s by the late Walter Bauer in Boston. At its opening, one of his hospital colleagues said to him 'Well, Walter, soon you will know everything about rheumatoid arthritis except its cause and cure.' Sadly, some years after his death that is still true.

Despite that nihilistic comment, much has changed about the way we can treat rheumatoid arthritis. When Marie Joseph first had rheumatoid arthritis we had two drugs, aspirin and gold, and there were few doctors

8

interested in the rheumatic diseases. Now we have twenty or thirty aspirin-like drugs, all of which we can use with relative safety to decrease the amount of swelling and pain in the joints, and lessen the dreadful morning and evening stiffness that affects the muscles. This means that we control symptoms in some 90 percent of the patients that we see with rheumatoid arthritis, an enormous advance on the late 1940s. During the first year or so of rheumatoid arthritis, approximately 40 percent of patients will have a spontaneous remission; in some never to recur and in others perhaps to have several more episodes in their life. Nowadays we watch patients with rheumatoid arthritis for at least two years, usually repeating the X-rays to check that there is no evidence of damage to the joints.

When damage is seen, or if we fail to control symptoms with non-steroidal drugs, we tend to use disease-modifying drugs, such as gold or penicillamine. These work more slowly and may have more side-effects, but in a large proportion of people they do control the disease and even make them asymptomatic. Another great advance for people unlucky enough to have severely damaged joints is that joint replacement – of many different types – is easier and safer.

Enormous advances have been made in the fields of 'why' and 'how' people develop rheumatoid arthritis. None is simple enough to allow us to understand the cause, or what the trigger is. We do know how the body mounts its attack on the joints and the other parts of the body. One day we may have a cure, but at present we have to be content with getting almost everybody better, if not as good as they were before the rheumatoid arthritis. The problem remains that none of the medications we use is perfect. All may have side-effects, some more than others. And in this day and age of information with the media so interested in medicine, almost everyone has heard of the awful side effects of this or that. Many people on their first consultation know more about

9

the side-effects that may happen than they realize how well we can control their illness. And everything, even crossing the road or changing a light-bulb in a ceiling light, has risks. Usually the side effects of a drug are not due to the drug. When drugs are developed, they are compared with an inactive tablet to show that they do work. And often the inactive tablet has the same number of side-effects!

One personal comment. The photograph of Marie Joseph on the original edition shows her with two sticks carefully hidden by the flowers. The flowers still bloom, but the sticks are no longer there.

J.M. Gumpel, F.R.C.P.
Consultant Physician and
Rheumatologist,
Northwick Park and
Mount Vernon Hospitals

# 1

I was brought up in a family so filled with stoicism that they would have made the Spartans seem like a bunch of raving hypochondriacs. My aunt had high blood-pressure, chronic bronchitis, and a heart that didn't beat as it should; but she would get up at seven o'clock every morning and cook our breakfast, coughing herself purple over the gas-stove, and sending me, and her own daughter Muriel, off to school with sore throats, pains in our legs – which she always dismissed as 'growing pains' – our necks bared to the cold Lancashire winds, because she said scarves over-heated the body.

The fact that I grew up at all must have justified her principles, because up to the age of seven, I had been a delicate and cosseted child, reared by a grandma (after my own mother had died having me) in an atmosphere redolent with liberty-bodices, tonic bottles from the doctor, opening medicines taken every Friday, and combinations worn winter and summer, which gave me a permanent itch where it was rude to scratch.

My hair was long and wavy, and the first thing my aunt did when I went to live with her after grandma died was to sit me on the piano stool, hand over her dressmaking scissors to my uncle, a mild-mannered, kindly man, and order him to cut off the lot.

I emerged looking like a moth-eaten lavatory brush, and stayed that way until well into adolescence.

The only time a visit to the doctor's surgery – a cheerless half of a terraced house, with horse-hair sofas and chairs oozing grey stuffing – was deemed necessary, was if we'd been running a temperature of 104° for a week, or if we'd fainted two days running.

We were great fainters, Muriel and I, usually in shops, and we took it in our strides, sitting passively outside the shop on a little hard chair, being wafted by someone's grocery list.

The doctor was called to the house only if our winter coughs began to resemble the death rattle . . .

So it was no wonder that when I fell downstairs and injured my wrist, so that a pain shot up my arm if I breathed on my little finger, I passed it off with a laugh known in romantic fiction as 'light'.

I was grown up by now, married, and living alone with my baby daughter, Marilyn, waiting for my husband Frank to come home after six years in the air force, three of them flying on operations.

The house we'd been lucky enough to rent was big and sparsely furnished. We had a tiny carpet in the dining-room, one utility sideboard, four ditto chairs, a square table, a bed upstairs, and a dressing-table and wardrobe so ugly, that even in those days of furniture dockets, they had stood unwanted in a second-hand shop for years.

Marilyn was a large and placid baby, nine months old, and still breast-fed.

'Anyone can breast feed,' my aunt had told me, and so I persevered, growing paler and thinner in the process, whilst the baby thrived and expanded in all directions. I was almost too scared to take her to the clinic, because the welfare lady, a round little body, with diamanté upsweeps to her spectacles, would tut-tut disapprovingly as I lowered my massive bundle on to the scales.

'A pound gain this week, Mother,' she'd say. 'Far too much. Six ounces at the most next week, now mind.'

And I'd say I'd try, but didn't know quite what to do, as all I was giving her was *me*. I hadn't seen my father since early childhood, but he was a big man, and so I put the blame on him.

The pram was a large and much handed-down model, and I became adept at pushing it with one hand after my fall downstairs, the pain in my right wrist when I tried to use it being bad enough to make me faint. Not that I ever did. With the passing of adolescence, and the responsibility of being a mother, fainting was a pastime I hadn't the urge to indulge in. I was an over-conscientious mother, I know that now. If the baby hadn't had her bath each evening, I felt I couldn't have answered for the consequences. To bath her in the huge and draughty bathroom was impossible. Those were the days when only the very rich had central heating, and anyway, I'd been conditioned over the years to freezing rooms, and been brain-washed into believing that an over-heated atmosphere was a harbinger of germs, and worse.

So, all alone, and nightly, I would stagger from the kitchen to the fire in the dining-room-cum-living room, the water in the bath tested by my elbow in the manner advocated in my baby manual, sloshing over the sides and wetting me through. Not being of a practical turn of mind, it never occurred to me to use a relay system of little jugs. I'd read so many books on how to bring up baby, I was an expert on the right colour of motions, and spent so long poking little swabs of cotton-wool up Marilyn's nose and down her ears, it's a wonder she didn't grow up devoid of the mucus membranes in all her orifices.

There was only enough coal for one fire, and even then I got a few bags on the black market. My coalman had failed his medical, and when all his mates were called up, took it upon himself to make his own deliveries. He was a beautiful man with a noble brow, very refined, and with an Oxford accent at complete and utter variance with the coal dust on his face. His vowels were so cultured, he made the word 'coal' sound like a two-syllabled musical cadence, not a black and filthy necessity, and when he'd dumped my ration in the outside shed – there was never any need to stand at the window counting the bags, as I'd been brought up to do, he being far too posh to cheat – he would lean against the kitchen door, discussing the vagaries of Marcel Proust, or the way Tennyson made his words sing, and when I paid him, I always felt I was insulting him in some indefinable way.

My wrist grew steadily more painful, and I developed twinges in my knees, but refused to acknowledge them, working on the theory that the human body can only cope with one pain at a time. I found a way of fastening a nappy with my left hand and my teeth, and discovered that opening doors, turning on taps, holding a pencil, became virtually impossible. Fortunately the bulk of my letter-writing came to an end when Frank was at last demobbed, and it was at his insistence that I took myself and my stubborn wrist to the village doctor.

He was a small square man with a nose much too big for his face – a lumpy mottled purple nose, which made me long to tell him about not drinking liquids too hot, and to ask him had he ever considered a dab of green powder? It took my attention from what I was trying to tell him, but something must have penetrated because he wrote a letter to the local infirmary, and made an appointment for me to see someone there and have an X-ray.

I didn't tell him about the twinges in my knees, or about the longing I had all day to lie down on the floor and sleep. I'd waited an hour and a half to see him, and the waiting-room was still full of people who looked and sounded much sicker than me. That part of Lancashire is noted for its dampness, hence the cotton mills, and the rows of terraced houses surrounding them, and it had seemed as I sat waiting my turn to go in that half the population must be suffering from a virulent form of advanced bronchitis, judging by the coughing and weary faces, so who was I to complain about a sprained wrist?

Apart from this, the very sight of a doctor sitting opposite to me, pen poised over his prescription pad, has

14

the effect of making me go into a Big Act. I get the same feeling that comes to old troupers when the overture sounds, and the curtains swish apart. It's as though by keeping my complaints to the minimum, I'm daring him to take me seriously. I have made more doctors laugh than I care to remember, and I know I must have been a welcome change from all the grey-faced moaners he sees in the course of one day. The plain fact that I must have misled a lot of them who haven't the time or the inclination to be psychiatrists has only recently occurred to me.

It was the same with the doctor at the Infirmary, an austere red-bricked building with echoing corridors, and flights of wide stone stairs. He couldn't have been long out of medical school, and he told me kindly that the X-ray had shown nothing broken, and suggested that they put my wrist in a splint for about six weeks or more.

'And who would bath my baby?' I said, laughing that one off, then told him, quite honestly, that it hadn't been so painful for the past few days.

He held my wrist, stared at it for a good five minutes, obviously puzzled. I expected him to reach at any moment for a medical book and look something up. There were two young nurses in the room at the time, and I saw them exchange a glance, an amused glance, and I felt sorry for him. He hadn't a clue as to what was wrong with my wrist, and bent it back experimentally. I smiled at him to show it didn't hurt, whilst waves of pain made even my arm-pits tingle.

'That hurt?' he asked me, and as his earnest face swam back into focus I assured him that it didn't, not much, not at all, really. That's another thing. I have an aversion to letting anyone see that I'm in pain, and fortunately I have a face that helps the illusion, round and chubby, with no interesting hollows, or pain-shadowed bags underneath my eyes. He tapped his teeth with a long black pencil, and came to a decision. 'Come and see me again in a month,' he said, and passed gratefully on to the next patient.

15

Now *she* walked in with an impressive limp, and looked as if she'd been dead for years, but couldn't summon up the sense to stiffen herself. I knew he'd find her far more satisfactory.

We got a baby-sitter for the next evening, and went out to a party. I arranged my hair with my left hand, telling myself firmly that of course I was just dying to go out; that of course I wouldn't prefer to go to bed with a good book. The party was being given by a teacher friend of mine and her husband, a serious couple whose idea of making a party go was to organize every single minute into playing games. Not for them, sitting around on cushions, talking, and listening to records. Angela, in her bossy teacher's voice split us into two teams, and started us off with a pencil and paper quiz.

'No cheating now!' she said, and I stared down at the list of questions, knowing with certainty that I was going to let my side down. One either has a quiz mind, or one hasn't, and I couldn't bring myself to *care* which was the odd man out, or what relation to each other two men in a tub were if one had an auntie who was stepmother to the other. What were they *doing* in a tub anyway?

So I wasn't surprised to find, when the totals were added up, that my marks were 10 out of a possible 105.

The winning team congratulated each other, and Angela marshalled us into two lines for the next game. This time we queued up behind our leader and, one by one, knelt down on the floor and wafted a tissue-paper fish along with a folded newspaper towards a chalked ring at the far end of the room. My team were actually jumping up and down with excitement because they were winning easily, and I tried hard to *care*. I tried not to let them down again, but when my turn came to kneel on the floor, the pain in my knees was so acute that I finished my stint bending over from the waist, praying that my utility knickers weren't showing, and fanning the flimsy fish along with my left hand, keeping my right wrist well tucked into my side. Needless to say the other team won, and I couldn't have felt more ashamed if I'd been competing in the team relay at the Olympic games, and had dropped the baton halfway round.

Angela's quick eyes missed nothing, and as she was the leader of my team, and feeling I'd let her down rather badly, I explained about my poor knees and sore wrist, making light of it, of course. She was such a bouncy girl, but with a heart as big as a football, and she put her arm round me.

'You know, love, I think you've got arthritis,' she said. 'I have an aunt who started just like you, with a fall. First her hands, then her knees, and within three years she was in a wheelchair. I think you should have a second opinion.'

It was a long walk home. Those were the days when cars were as thick on the ground as snow in August, and it seemed to me that my shoes had suddenly shrunk until they were three sizes too small. I had in fact mentioned this to my aunt before, and she'd said that everybody's feet swelled in summer.

But this was October, a cold starless night, with the first touch of frost in the air. In rather a small voice, not wishing to alarm him, I told Frank about Angela and her second opinion, and to my surprise, he immediately said he thought she was right.

'You haven't been looking yourself lately,' he said kindly, and I trudged on, every step now a burning agony, a clear picture in my mind of myself in a wheelchair, the basket type you could lie down in, being pushed down a road, with a red blanket encompassing me from chin to ankles, and passers-by making sympathetic clucking noises over me: 'So young to be struck down like that in her prime.'

The next day, pegging nappies out awkwardly with my left hand, I tried out Angela's theory on my next-door neighbour, a grey-haired little body, having a terrible time with her menopause.

'A friend thinks I have arthritis,' I said, making it

17

sound like I thought it was the joke of the year.

She perked up no end. 'I had an uncle with that. He spent the last ten years of his life in bed, wrapped from head to foot in cotton wool. The only part of him that moved was his eyeballs.'

I went inside the house, and leaned against the sink, seeing a clear vision of myself swathed in layers of cotton wool, passing on urgent and frantic messages to my long-suffering family, with jerky twitchings of my eyelids. Then Marilyn started to cry, and I went to pick her up, feeling the now all too familiar pain shoot up my arm as I held her awkwardly against my shoulder. Her Friar Tuck fringe of hair was black with sweat, and her mouth was a round O of indignation as she screamed for her feed. I sat down, unfastened my blouse, and watched her eyes roll in ecstasy as she began to suck vigorously. I saw her childhood stretching ahead, marred and spoilt by caring for an invalid mother. I saw her rushing home from school to tuck me more comfortably into my cotton-wool cocoon, and I saw her struggling to interpret the pathetic little messages relayed by my swivelling eyeballs . . . .

The next day I went back to the village doctor, and trying not to stare at his nose, made a clean breast of *all* my symptoms, and asked him outright for a second opinion.

An appointment was fixed for me to see an eminent specialist in Manchester. There was no National Health Service in those days, and we could ill afford the five guinea fee. My mother-in-law offered to take care of the baby, saying a bottle feed wouldn't harm her for once, and my aunt said she would come with me to Manchester, as she wanted to look round for a winter coat. She had always been a great one for killing two birds with one stone, and when I told her I might have rheumatoid arthritis, she merely sniffed. 'Everybody in our family has rheumatism,' she said, and I could have kissed her. 'Look at your auntie Mabel and her feet, and

18

your auntie Ethel and her back, and no wonder. When we used to stand at our looms in the mill when we were girls, our feet were always in running damp. Our house smelt of wintergreen winter and summer, and your grandma had rheumatism round her heart. That didn't kill her though,' she added hastily.

Outside the station in Manchester we caught a tram out to the labyrinth of posh streets where all the eminent specialists practised. I wasn't to know it at the time, but the man I was going to see was knighted for his services in the field of rheumatism in the next few years, so that shows just how eminent he was. He was big and burly and hairy, just like a bear, and my automatic act of nonchalance didn't fool him, not one little bit.

'You have rheumatoid arthritis,' he told me simply, after a brief examination. 'There is no known cure as yet, but rest and warmth, and pain-killing drugs will all play their part.' Then, just for a moment, he placed a huge hand on my shoulder. 'You have a tough time ahead, my dear, but sometimes this thing burns itself out, and this is what we hope will happen in your case. Stick to a good nourishing diet, plenty of protein, and try not to worry. The emotions play no part in the onset of arthritis, but a great part in the way you can face up to it. I'll write to your doctor, and he will keep an eye on you.'

I got dressed again, thanked him, handed over the five guinea fee to his receptionist, and joined my aunt in the beautifully furnished waiting-room.

'I've got it,' I said, and she sniffed.

'So have most people, and there's a lot of worse things you could be having, and now we'll have a spot of lunch, and start off at C & A. I don't see the point of paying fancy prices, when some of their things are just as nice.'

Her attitude wasn't all that I could have hoped for, but it was the right one, I'm sure of that. She knew I had a tendency to over-dramatize myself, plus an imagination which needed tight reins on it. In the restaurant she chose a salad for her figure, but I chose eggs on toast

19

because of the protein, and as I ate I was worrying about how I was going to feed myself on steaks, when Frank's take-home pay was exactly £3. ls. 8d., twenty-eight shillings of which went on rent for the big house we'd been lucky to get. He was finishing off his studies at Technical College for two days each week, plus three evenings at night school, and he was discovering, like so many other men who had spent six years away at the war, that now he was back he could expect no concessions. That he was, in fact, to be penalized for helping us to win the war.

It was late afternoon when we caught the train back home, my aunt sitting flushed and satisfied with the huge paper bag containing her coat on the seat beside her, and me so exhausted that I forgot about catching things in my hair from the upholstery and leant back with my eyes closed. My breasts hurt with their accumulation of milk, and I felt a sense of complete anti-climax. I'd been told I had a dreadful disease. It *was* a dreadful disease, it said so in my *Home Doctor*, and I felt I should have been sent back home in a white ambulance, bells ringing, and blue lights flashing on top, being put straight to bed, with cotton wool instead of sheets, and all my friends and relatives tiptoeing in to stand at the foot of my bed, staring at me, and talking in whispers.

Instead of that I rushed round to my mother-in-law's house, just round the corner from where we lived, collected the baby, and in between bathing her – it never occurred to me to give that routine a miss for one day – I managed to get a shepherd's pie in the oven. I was tired halfway to death, and one knee had swollen up in sympathy, or was it just to prove the eminent specialist right? But of one thing I was certain.

I wasn't going to give in to it. My little family wasn't going to suffer, just because I was suffering. Marilyn would grow up as well cared for, as cherished, as if her mother was in the rudest of health, with muscles of steel. I wouldn't complain, I wouldn't moan. Good for a laugh

20

I'd always been, and good for a laugh I'd be from now on. Pollyanna would be like a real old misery compared to me.

And with that nauseating picture in my mind, I staggered upstairs with the baby, lowered her painfully into her drop-sided cot, went back downstairs into the kitchen, and with my left hand whipped up a sponge for the baked apple pudding.

# 2

Being an arthritic is a deflating thing to be, a one in the eye to the ego. It creeps up on you insidiously, and knowing that you are probably going to have it for the rest of your life means that you can't, even right at the beginning, make the most of it.

It's not *romantic*. I don't remember one heroine, in all the books I've read, who had arthritis. Camille could be seen daintily touching a lace-edge handkerchief to her mouth without upsetting anyone overmuch, and even leukaemia has been recently glamorized in books and on the screen. I actually read one novel where the hero was a leper, but of course he walked away into the jungle before things started dropping off. I suppose it's partly because arthritis is not a fatal disease, and partly because the treatment for it is not conducive to romance. What man is there who would want to plight his troth to a woman who sits with her feet in a bowl of epsom-salted water four times a day? Or to one who can't get her right arm high enough to wind it lovingly around his neck?

During that first year, I stuck to my avowed intention of carrying on regardless, improvising like mad when ordinary domestic tasks proved to be beyond me.

Both hands were by now swollen, misshapen, and extremely painful. Combing and brushing my shoulder-length hair was a frustrating, hopeless task, so I had it cut off, and wore it in the very short bubble-cut style made famous by Ingrid Bergman in the film *For Whom the Bell Tolls*. The effect wasn't quite the same, but it made life much easier. I found out I could fasten my bra by the simple expedient of hooking it up at the front, then swivelling it round. But fastening my suspenders to my stockings (this was before the glorious advent of tights) became a sweating, hazardous process.

One Sunday morning in church, as we sang the first hymn, I felt my left stocking sliding down my leg, and as it was a Communion service, and I would be in view as I limped up to the altar rail, I managed, during a prayer, to unfasten the other side, and allowed that stocking to slide down to match.

We bought a third-hand bicycle, and I found I could ride when walking was impossible, so I pedalled to and from the shops, leaving Marilyn sleeping in her pram in the garden under the eye of my kindly neighbour. With my short-cropped hair and round face, I presented a picture of blooming health as I cycled along. And that was what seemed to matter . . . .

When Marilyn was just over two years old, I told Frank it was time we had another baby.

'I'm going to have arthritis perhaps for the rest of my life,' I said, 'And if I want an excuse for not having another baby, I've got one. But we always said we'd have two at least, and I'll get through, I know I will. I've read that arthritic symptoms may disappear when a woman's pregnant, so for that alone it's worth considering.'

We were young, and incredibly optimistic. There had been a war, hadn't there, and we'd come through that? So, no sooner said than done, and William (for of course this time it was going to be a boy) was on his way.

And like a miracle, just as the book had said they might, my arthritic symptoms virtually disappeared. I am one of those irritating women who blossom when they're pregnant. No early morning sickness, cramps, piles, varicose veins, lank hair, peculiar food fads, troubled me. Contrary to all I read in my *Home Doctor*, I never once yearned for pickled cabbage in the middle of the night, never went off my husband, suffered from feelings of panic, gloom, either pre- or post-natal; just as now, well through the menopause, I still wait in vain for my first hot flush.

'I'll just have to keep on having babies, one after the other,' I told the doctor at the clinic, as he checked me over for high blood-pressure and worse, and found me singularly lacking.

He lacked a sense of humour. 'You're going to need help when this baby arrives,' he told me, shaking his head sadly as he held my right hand, with its sloping fingers and protruding knuckles. 'Nature is merely giving you a respite, my dear.'

I knew I had to cheer him up. There were fourteen heavily pregnant women in the cheerless waiting-room, and I was sure the sight of all those enlarged stomachs and jutting navels was making him morose. It showed in his face. He had long, drooping jowls, like a blood-hound, his white coat was unfastened to reveal a grey cardigan with pockets in the regions of his knee-caps. He was coming up to retirement, I guessed, and a lifetime of peering up women's vaginas in the surroundings of the bleak hospital was enough to take the joy out of any man's life. So I smiled at him.

'*My* arthritis isn't going to come back,' I told him confidently. 'I'm a biological phenomenon, didn't you know? You'll be able to write me up in the *Lancet*.

He wasn't impressed.

'The baby's head hasn't engaged yet, so I suggest you come in in a month's time, two weeks before it's due, and we'll induce, then if you need a Caesarean, I'll be around to give you one.'

'Thank you, but I'm sure that won't be necessary,' I told him. But he wasn't listening, and the nurse in charge, a vehement middle-aged tartar with a moustache and a face that looked as it it would disintegrate if she smiled, motioned for me to get down from the high bed, and make room for the next patient.

The hospital, high on a hill, was an austere, splayed-out collection of buildings that had formerly been the workhouse. Dickens would have loved it and I could imagine queues of dispirited down-and-outs lining the long bare corridors with their little bowls in their hands, patiently waiting for their dollop of grey gruel. The bottom half of the walls was painted a shiny bottle-green, whilst the top half glowed a bilious shade of yellow. There was a demarcation line in brown dividing the two, and the whole effect was so hideous that I could only conclude that those responsible had bought up the paint in a huge lot for practically nothing. There were twenty to thirty beds in each ward, and as I walked back towards the main door, I could see each bed 'dressed' in line, the faded pink bedspreads tucked in with uncompromising hospital precision.

I didn't want our William to be born in such a setting. I'd imagined myself sitting up in bed at home, surrounded by flowers and friends, with him lying in a frilled treasure-cot, and Marilyn bending over him, like an illustration in a glossy magazine. Being an arthritic hadn't done a thing for my ego, but having a baby was going to restore at least some of my flagging confidence. I wasn't going to lie in one of those beds, staring at those horrible yellow and green walls. Not if I could help it!

The date fixed for me to be admitted was 31 January, a Saturday, the day my doctor kept aside for his Caesareans, and I went by myself in a taxi, Frank staying home to take care of Marilyn.

That in itself was an occasion, taxis only being used in my family for weddings and funerals. The driver had an over-developed sense of the dramatic, and after seeing my bulging stomach, exceeded the speed-limit the whole way. He was so obviously enjoying himself, I hadn't the heart to tell him I was merely keeping an appointment. When he wasn't actually engaged in turning a corner on two wheels, he would look over his shoulder, and enquire: 'All right, love?' For his sake I tried to look as if my pains were coming thick and fast, and we turned into the vast gravel forecourt of the hospital stopping with a lurch that almost sent me catapulting over the back of the seat and through the windscreen.

The doctor who had been detailed to induce me, was tall and fair and very young, with a most engaging manner. I don't know whether inducing a baby nowadays is a more refined procedure, but in those days, the way they did it wasn't guaranteed to make a woman feel at her most alluring. The bottom half of the bed was removed, whilst the patient's legs were tethered high and wide apart. The induction itself was perfectly painless, being a breaking of the waters to bring on labour, and as the handsome doctor came towards me, smiling pleasantly, remarking how cold the weather was, even for the time of the year, I turned my face into my pillow and closed my eyes, my conversational technique with doctors deserting me completely. Concluding I was deaf, I suppose, he went away, his little task completed, and left me to the ministrations of a pint-sized nurse with flaming red hair and freckles, and the name of Kelly. She took me through into one of the huge wards, and I climbed into a bed with a sag-in-the-middle mattress, and the loudspeaker for the radio right above my head. I lay there in my uncomfortable hollow, hoping Frank had remembered how to light the inside of the oven. A pink bedjacket in the next bed leaned over and told me she had been in labour for three whole days, was forty-four and had thought that her baby was 'the change' until the onset of her pains, which even then she'd dismissed as the result of a tin of plums which had blown.

Watching the wobbling of her three chins as she spoke, I could well believe it. That evening, after the longest day of my life, a little bald-headed man came and sat by her bed and held her hand, and talked non-stop about the miracle of their baby, and it was beautiful . . . .

The night nurses came on duty, and gave me something to drink which looked and tasted like thick brown gear oil. Not liking to tell them that three aspirins are enough to send me into a coma, so much do I over-react to drugs, I swallowed it down obediently and went into a deep sleep, to wake up in the labour ward with a nurse telling me to hold my breath as the baby's head was being born.

Two years afterwards, when I was in the same hospital being treated for arthritis, the same nurse was to tell me that I was the only woman she had ever known who had literally had her baby in her sleep.

'Were you very close to your mother?' she asked me.

'She died having me,' I told her.

The nurse nodded, well satisfied. 'She had the baby for you, my dear,' she said.

I was more intrigued than convinced, but it was certainly a beautiful idea.

And William, who turned out to be Katy, was a perfect doll of a wee thing. She was so pretty, I could feel only pity for the other mothers when their babies, pale and pallid, were brought in to be fed. She had soft brown hair, upward slanting dark eyes, and a gorgeous sunburnt complexion. Nurse Kelly told me it was jaundice because she was premature, but I refused to listen even when, on my return home, she turned bright yellow.

The arthritis came back as I lay in bed for the two weeks deemed necessary in those days. My ankles refused to revert to walking position when I tried to stand up, and my hands swelled so much that to dress my baby left me weak and trembling with frustration. I was allocated a home help, and a district nurse who came daily to bath the baby, and we found Mrs Cronshawe, who came twice weekly to do what she called the 'rough'.

The house teemed with domestics, but nothing seemed to get done. They hated each other on sight, and the mornings when the three of them were in the house at once, tripping over each other, exhausted me to the point when every nerve in my body seemed to be alive and jangling.

The home help explained to me kindly that she wasn't supposed to do the washing; Mrs Cronshawe explained that because of her dizzy spells, she couldn't reach above her head, or stoop to clean anything at floor level, and the district nurse took one look at the baby bath and asked for the washing-up bowl, and told me that the cot, by our bed, was in a howling draught.

And three weeks after I'd settled back home, Marilyn developed measles.

The spots took a long time to come out, and I had put her tantrums, refusal to eat, and constant demand for attention down to the fact that she was jealous of her new little sister. The very morning I called in the doctor, she had been leaning over the cot, coughing on the baby, and when I asked him if she was likely to get it, he fingered his bumpy nose.

'Let's just say we sincerely hope not,' he said.

'Do *you* think she'll get it?' I asked Mrs Cronshawe, the home help having departed in high dudgeon because of something the district nurse was supposed to have said.

'If she does I dread to think how a wee skinned rabbit as she is will ever stand the fever,' said Mrs C.

The district nurse merely told me to keep them well apart.

I went into action, as detailed in my *Home Doctor*, hanging a Dettol-soaked sheet over the door of Marilyn's room, and frightening the baby out of her tiny mind by giving her her bottle with a home-made yashmak tied round my face that made it almost impossible to breathe. In those days, measles cases were kept in darkened rooms, the curtains tightly drawn to keep out the light, supposed to be bad for their eyes, and I spent anxious days tottering from one child to the other, carefully scrubbing my poor aching hands each time. I never see a bottle of Dettol nowadays without remembering . . . .

Katy didn't get the measles, and someone told us about this marvellous little man at the other end of town.

He was an osteopath, faith-healer, physiotherapist and miracle-worker combined, apparently, so on one of the days when Frank came home early from Technical College, I caught the bus and went to be faith-healed or whatever.

His waiting room was his parlour, an over-stuffed room, with display cabinets filled with bric-à-brac, plaster birds flying in frantic trios round the speckled walls, a herd of pottery elephants trudging across the mantelpiece, four china bunnies squatting in a row on the tiled hearth, and bits of chintz covering the chintz covers on the settee and chairs.

'Suffered with my back for years,' the man in the next chair to me was telling the man in the next chair to him. 'Slept on a door for five years, and had to give it up . . . .' Here his voice sank to a whisper, but it wasn't hard to imagine what he'd sacrificed. I was trying so hard to eavesdrop, I was sure my left ear was flapping. 'Then I came to see Mr Woolley, and one click and I was cured. I come regular like once a month, just for a going-over, and he fairly puts me through it, but it's worth it.'

'You've got arthritis, haven't you, love?' the woman on my other side was saying. 'I noticed your hands the minute you came in.'

I looked down at my hands, and tried in vain to hold them in a more natural position. I had asked Frank many times if they were noticeable, and he'd sworn on his very life that it was impossible for anyone to see the slightest abnormality in them. I'd almost believed him too, because I wanted to believe him. For the first time the word 'deformed' flashed across my mind, and I felt that everyone in that crammed little room was staring at me. I would have sat on the offenders if it wouldn't have hurt too much, and I made an unkept vow to wear mittens from then on, and never do anything that would draw attention to them.

'My mother-in-law had it,' my friend on my right was saying. 'Her hands were so crippled, she had to do all her housework with the tips of her little fingers. Pitiful to see her it was. Have you got any children, love?'

'Two little girls,' I told her, 'but I can do everything for them. Everything.'

Sadly she disillusioned me. 'If I were you, love, I'd train them to be independent as soon as you can. It's a cruel thing, arthritis is.'

She pronounced it 'authoritis', and I hated her. I turned my back on her, and tried to hear further revelations from the man on my left, the sexually frustrated one who'd spent five years on a door. I was discovering how hard it was to keep up my own morale in the face of the pessimistic outlook of so many people who were genuinely sorry for me, and only trying to be kind and sympathize.

'Walking badly today, aren't you, love?' my neighbour would say as I limped past her gate. If only she could have said, 'Walking better today,' what a difference it would have made. Even Pollyanna herself, I concluded, would have been hard put to it at times to see the bright side of things . . . .

I was so depressed by the time I went in to see Mr Woolley, the miracle-worker, that I abandoned my usual jollying-up-the-doctor act, and told him about my aching hands, knees, ankles, shoulders, and threw in the recent pains at the top of my spine, and the difficulty in chewing my food for good measure.

Mr Woolley was a good man. Goodness was written in every line of his Gentle Jesus type of face. He didn't tell me to climb up on his examination couch; instead he leaned forward and took both my hands in his own.

'I'm going to be honest with you, love,' he said. 'I'm a quack with a knack of putting bones back where they belong when they've slipped out of place. Show me a disc out of place, and I can manipulate it quicker than you can say Jack Knife.'

'One click and I'd be cured,' I said, quoting the man on the door, and he smiled.

'But arthritis when it's flared-up, like yours is at the moment, I daren't touch, wouldn't be right. This is something you have to come to terms with, love. But I can tell you right here and now, that I've known many cases burn themselves out, and that's what I hope will happen to you. And you know, however bad the pain is, you don't die with arthritis.'

'I told a neighbour that,' I said.

'And what did she say?' asked dear kind, saintly Mr Woolley.

'The more's the pity,' I said, and left him laughing, and refusing to take his usual fee – five shillings.

Katy was crying for her bottle when I arrived back home, and Frank was trying to study with her tucked underneath one arm. I went into the kitchen, without stopping to take off my coat, and as I lifted the heavy pan I kept for boiling up her bottles in, the whole thing slipped from my awkward grasp and crashed to the floor, scattering teats and bottles, and spreading water over the linoleum. The noise woke Marilyn, who had taken lately to climbing out of her single bed and coming downstairs to see what she might be missing.

She stood there in the kitchen doorway, a matronly little figure, her two short plaits sticking out on each side of her round face, thumb in mouth, whilst behind her Frank hovered, a damp screaming baby and a textbook tucked underneath his arm.

I knelt down painfully on one knee, trying to clean up the mess, with fingers too stiff and swollen to do my bidding, and I wondered what would have happened if I'd followed my instincts, thrown myself flat among the debris, and burst into self-pitying tears.

Then I saw the little circle of faces watching me anxiously, and my aunt's voice came to me telling me once that the whole happiness of any family depended on the mood of the mother. If she was sad, then they were sad also; if she smiled and made the best of things, then so did they. It was as simple as that.

So I laughed, and they laughed with me. At least my husband and elder daughter laughed. Nothing would have pacified the screaming bundle of fury tucked in an unnatural position underneath his arm.

So I picked up a bottle, rinsed it underneath the tap, and got on with mixing her feed. Pollyanna had triumphed once again . . . .

# 3

Having arthritis in its acute form, and with two small children to look after in a large and draughty house, is a bit like trying to climb Mount Everest in winkle-pickers. There are some days when you don't get very far.

The complaint flits – a medical term, not mine – from joint to joint, with dogged persistence. You come to terms with not being able to use a hand properly, then wake up one morning to find that your big toe joints are so swollen that you cannot bear to wear even the softest of bedroom slippers.

It does, however, ensure that you never become a *bore*. If asked how you are, and you are foolish enough to answer truthfully, there is always a different part to complain about.

I learnt quite early to answer 'fine' every time my health was enquired about, and I'm sure that was the way I kept my friends, and ensured the sanity of my family. 'How d'you do?' is one of the most hypocritical phrases in the English language. No one really wants to know how you do, however much they may love you; they have their own lives to be getting on with, and I've never been able to convince myself that pity is all that much akin to love . . . .

By the time Katy was a few months old, the district nurse and the home help had gone their separate ways, and we found we could no longer afford Mrs Cronshawe to do our rough, so I was entirely on my own.

And whereas Marilyn had been a placid baby, doing

everything according to the book, Katy was a born rebel. She slept for short periods during the day, and for part of the evening, but when Frank and I went to bed – that was the time she came into her own, as they say in that part of Lancashire.

She spent many happy hours sandwiched in between Frank and me in our double bed, very often upside down, her damp little bottom up against my face – damp, in spite of three thicknesses of nappies, because only careless mothers put their babies in rubber pants in those days before the advent of plastic pants. And down in the bed, up against our feet, was her night feed, a bottle made up hot, wrapped in a clean towel and small blanket, and fished up when her screams became so demanding that they couldn't be ignored.

My wrists by now were so swollen and painful that I couldn't hold the bottle in the normal way, and I devised a method whereby I rested it against the pillow, and clamped her on to it, whilst Frank slept peacefully on.

Round about the time when dawn began to crack, I became adept at dropping her over the side of her cot, the small hinges being beyond my manipulation, and then I would sleep so heavily that on quite a few occasions, Frank would wake me up, just to reassure himself that I was still alive.

The only medication I was taking was aspirins, even now thought to be more than the equal of any of the modern so-called wonder drugs, but many and varied were the 'cures' suggested to me by well-meaning relatives and friends.

I tried them all.

The cabbage leaves tied round my knees when I went to bed, making me smell like a compost heap when I got warm. Honey swallowed by the bucketful, especially queen bee's. The hot poultices slapped on until my joints blistered; and the cold ones, making my skin redden in angry protest. The herb tea that someone's Auntie Annie had cured herself with in three weeks flat, and the salts (enough to cover a sixpenny-piece) taken first thing in a cup of warm water. My symptoms didn't disappear, but I must have had the cleanest intestines that side of the Pennines.

The piece of potato carried around in my apron pocket, the copper bracelet worn on my wrist, and the cider apple vinegar drunk with every meal, ruining the taste of the food and making me screw up my face into what Frank said was a horrible grimace with every sip.

And, oh, the beautiful, positive thoughts I wallowed in! I read all about the power of mind over matter, and I told myself my arthritis was all in the mind. It *didn't* hurt to walk, and I *could* raise my right arm, and as for my hands, they were the shape they were simply because I was being negative, and not trying hard enough.

I loved everyone, I encompassed my whole world in a wave of blind adoration, and every night before I went to sleep, I told myself firmly that I was absolutely rude with health, and that when I awoke I would leap from my bed, and run around the way I used to do.

And nothing worked.

But the girls grew out of babyhood, Frank passed more exams, and when Marilyn was four she went to school. It was two painful years after that, when turning over in bed one night, I slightly dislocated a wobbly knee joint, and the doctor told me that I ought to go into hospital for a period of bed-rest. Two months at least, he said.

'Impossible,' I told him. 'I could never leave my family, not for that length of time. What would become of them?'

He had kind eyes, and he talked to me as if he really cared. As if he were my father.

'What kind of a mother are you going to be if you become completely crippled?' he asked me. 'You are only a step away from a wheelchair as it is. Rest is the only thing that will help you now. Think it over, my dear . . .'

Frank had borrowed his father's car to run me to the hospital for the consultation, and we sat outside in one of the little side streets whilst I told him what the doctor had said.

I remember a girl walked past, a child clinging to either hand. A girl walking with a springy step, her hair tossing on her shoulders as she went, and I thought about my own slow shuffle, and how my girls had never known the joy of having a mother who could run with them, and for the first time since I'd been told I had arthritis, I broke down and cried self-pitying tears.

Frank was so astonished, I don't think he knew quite what to do. I *never* cried. I was the one who faced up to things. I *hated* people who indulged in self-pity. I'd said so, over and over again.

He patted my shoulder, handed me his handkerchief, and told me to blow, and I said I was sorry, and that I wasn't crying because I had arthritis, but because I was going to leave them for a long time, and because I didn't know what they were going to do.

'We'll think of something,' said Frank, and that evening, with the girls in bed, we sat round the living-room fire and talked; and when we went to bed we were certain of one thing. Somehow they would stay together, the three of them; there was to be no question of the girls being separated, or leaving their home. The next day we went along to see the vicar.

Did he know, we asked him, of any woman in the village who would come each morning from Monday to Friday, as Frank left for work, to see Marilyn off to school, and stay until he came home at six o'clock? Frank, with his engineering qualifications to back him up, had been promoted, and we could afford to pay £3 a week. We had a washing machine, I explained, and I couldn't help the note of pride in my voice as I thought about it.

It was a cumbersome thing, and had to be dragged up to the sink and filled with hot water from the tap. There

36

was a handle attachment on the top, and you moved it by hand backwards and forwards, so that it agitated the clothes, then you let out the soapy water by turning on a little tap at the bottom, and filled it up again with rinsing water. When it was first delivered, I just stood and stared at it, considering myself to be the luckiest woman alive. It wasn't until I'd used it for the first time, and discovered that working the handle put my wrists out of action, that we decided to wash on Sunday mornings. I did everything but actually motivate the handle. Frank would stand there, smoking a cigarette and reading the Sunday paper, working the handle furiously backwards and forwards, and trying hard not to look as if he was domesticated. There were certain jobs he would willingly help me with, but not if they challenged his masculinity. Dusting was out, drying the dishes was out, but washing them didn't emasculate him too much. He would even mop the kitchen floor if needs be, but only from a stooping position – never on his knees. Frying bacon and eggs was OK, but lighting the inside of the oven and putting a casserole in was sissy. He would press his own trousers and iron his ties, but running the iron over a pillowcase was definitely out. And now I was going to have to go away, and leave him to the ministrations of some unknown woman who wouldn't understand how he felt about such things . . . .

The vicar, a slight, fair, intellectual young man with an Adam's apple which bobbed up and down as he spoke, said he'd try to help. He thought he knew the very person who would fit our requirements, a Mrs Barlowe, recently widowed, who was seventy-one, clean and thoroughly trustworthy. He would go and see her the very next day, he promised, the Adam's apple working convulsively, and told us that the Lord would see us through.

We walked home slowly and collected the children from our next-door neighbour. After they'd gone to bed, I watched Frank get out his books, then I got out my knitting believing, quite wrongly as it happened, that knitting kept the fingers going.

As I struggled with a pattern row, I was wondering if the unknown Mrs Barlowe would understand that when Katy was feverish she needed the old grey blanket, referred to as her suck-a-blanket, to take everywhere with her, one corner of it wrapped around her fingers, as she sucked her thumb.

Would she understand that Marilyn wasn't surly and sulky when she refused to chat, but just pathologically shy? Did she know how to plait hair? And would she try to make Marilyn eat fish, which she loathed, or Katy cheese, which made her sick?

I was just nine years away from discovering that I had a gift, a flair, call it what you will, for writing short stories, and my first effort, typed on foolscap paper in single spacing, sold to the first magazine I sent it to. Now I know why; then I thought it was just a happy accident. It sold because it was about a mother who had to go into hospital, leaving her children behind, and it was written, as all the best stories are, right from the heart, and some kind editor, way up in Dundee, recognized this immediately.

The vicar called the next day, bringing Mrs Barlowe with him, and as soon as I saw her, I knew that the Lord was indeed on our side. She was stout and homely, with surprisingly black hair and short-sighted eyes which regarded me steadily from behind the whirlpool lenses of her spectacles.

I introduced her to the children.

'This is Mrs Barlowe,' I told Marilyn, who immediately narrowed her dark eyes into patronizing slits and retreated into one of her silences, which I knew from experience, nothing could break.

'This is Katy,' I told Mrs Barlowe, adding underneath my breath, 'they're very shy, I'm afraid, especially with strangers. . . .'

But Katy had seen the large mole growing out of Mrs

Barlowe's chin, with the single hair sprouting from it, and she put her head on one side, the way she always did before coming out with one of her more personal remarks. I'd told her firmly that it was very rude and unkind to say anything about another's face or person, and young as she was, she'd got the message, because the next time an aunt visited us, Katy had leaned against her chair, smiling at her and enquiring sweetly:

'*Some* ladies have moustaches, haven't they?'

A generalization, not a personal remark; even a two-year-old was astute enough to know that . . . .

I started to say something quickly, but in that split second Katy's attention had been distracted by the vicar's hassock.

'My daddy doesn't wear a black nightie,' she said, an observation far less loaded than references to hairy moles, and the moment had passed.

I showed Mrs Barlowe round the house, and explained that as there were no roads to cross, Marilyn could walk by herself to school. I showed her the washing-machine, and she sniffed.

'I'd rather dab-wash,' she said, so I agreed to the sheets and Frank's shirts going to the laundry, doing little sums in my mind as I talked, and praying that our budget would stretch that far. It was arranged that she would come in the following Monday, the day before I went into hospital. I thanked her and said I hoped she wouldn't find it all too much for her, when all I was wanting to say was:

'Just *love* them, that's all. Let the house drip with cobwebs, fluff collect underneath the beds, and ash pile up in the grate, but leave time for loving, please, please, please.'

Pretty speeches don't come easy in that part of Lancashire. Women like Mrs Barlowe had known two world wars, and a depression in between. With husbands on the dole, they had kept their terraced houses sparkling clean, and knew a pride so fierce it was almost terrifying.

'I'll watch out for 'em, love,' she said as she walked flat-footed down the path, and that was enough . . . more than enough.

That weekend I shopped, loading the push-chair with tins of corned beef, thick soups, things I would never have bought normally, but all in deference to Frank's aversion to cooking. I tried to make him take a lesson in omelette making, but knew he wasn't listening.

'We'll manage,' he kept saying. 'Just you go and get yourself put right,' but I made out little lists, and wore myself into a state of utter exhaustion by washing everything washable in the house, even Katy's suck-a-blanket, only to be told indignantly that it didn't smell right now!

I told the girls calmly and smilingly that Mummy was going away for a while, and that when I came back I would be able to run.

'And skip?' asked Marilyn, having mastered the art herself, just the week before.

'And skip,' I promised firmly.

Katy said nothing, just clung to me for the rest of the day, actually hanging on to my skirt, even waiting on the landing outside the lavatory until I came out.

'Three and a bit is the worst time of all to leave a child,' I told Frank. 'It could cause irreparable damage. Make her lose her sense of security. I can't go, it's impossible, can't you see?'

'You've read that in a book,' said Frank, and walked away from me, and not for the first time I marvelled at his practical turn of mind, his unflappable common sense, and thought how good he was for me.

Once again he borrowed his father's car, and took a couple of hours off work to drive me to the hospital. It was the same hospital where Katy had been born, but now, since the advent of the National Health, many changes had been made. The wards were still far too big, but the faded bedspreads had been replaced by bright blue covers, and the colour scheme was mauve and grey instead of the former bilious yellow and sickly green.

A nurse whisked me and my case away from Frank, and I tried hard to keep up with her as she walked briskly in a crackle of starched apron down the long corridor. She led me into a ward with twenty beds in it, ten down each side, and my first impression was that all the patients had died quietly without anyone noticing.

Grey heads and grey faces on stark white pillows; and the smell, in spite of the over-riding one of antiseptic, of old, old age. Not knowing quite what to do with me, I suppose, they'd put me into a kind of geriatric ward, and as I undressed behind tall screens, and the crackly nurse stored my dressing-gown and slippers away in the locker, I heard a low moaning wail from the next bed.

'Doris?' the plaintive voice was crying. 'Doris . . . Doris?'

The nurse took no notice, just went on folding the clothes up as I took them off and putting them back into the case.

'Doris . . . ?' came the anguished wail from the other side of the screen.

'Somebody wants Doris,' I said, resorting as usual to flippancy, because I was scared, and the nurse nodded.

'Poor old soul fell downstairs, and lay there for two days and nights before she was found. Doris is her niece,' she explained.

Then she pulled back the sheets and motioned for me to climb in, tucked me in so firmly that I felt I'd never see my arms again, whisked away the screens, and was gone. I turned my head, and saw a hawk-like nose above the sheet, a cloud of snow-white hair, and a thin hand working convulsively in the air as if trying to grasp something just out of reach.

'Doris . . .' the thin voice cried again, and I turned my head the other way, and saw in the next bed a pair of bird-bright eyes staring at me.

I started to sit up.

'No sitting up. No talking. It's the hour we have to rest,' the old lady told me in a voice so loud I was sure it would be heard in the next ward. 'What have they got you in for?'

'Arthritis,' I whispered, and by the way the beady eyes followed the movements of my lips, I realized the old lady was very deaf, and couldn't hear the sound of her own penetrating voice.

'Whereabouts?' she shouted.

'All over, I'm afraid.'

She immediately brightened up.

'See that lady in the far bed, the one with the cage over her legs, and the bedclothes held up with those little pegs? She's got arthritis, but hers has gone septic, poor thing. They have to feed her and do everything for her. How old are you, love? Eighteen?'

'I'm thirty-one.'

Two rows of sparkling white dentures clicked sympathetically.

'See that lady across? She's had a stroke, and lost the use of everything. I'm in here for my bowels. Perforated. Yes, every inch. Before I came in here, I had to . . .'

Then followed an exact description of the precise course her complaint had taken, and as she went into nauseating detail, I felt the cold hand of horror squeeze my heart, which was thumping so hard I was sure the old lady on my right would hear it.

But she was past hearing anything.

'Doris?' she called. 'Doris?'

It was as though I had suddenly been plunged into a nightmare, or found myself part of a horror film come to life. If a doctor had come through the swing doors with a bolt through his neck, I wouldn't have turned a hair. I was ill, I was really sick. That was why they'd put me in this ward with all these obviously terminal cases. I didn't know that arthritis could go septic, but apparently it could. I was doomed. Frank would marry again, of course. He was very attractive to women, I knew. He would mourn me of course, for a while . . . . I saw him being led away from my graveside, with the two little

42

girls dressed all in black, with black ribbon bows on their plaits.

I sat up in bed, just as a young and incredibly handsome young doctor, his white coat flying, came through the door. He charged down the long ward, saw me, and came to a skidding full stop by my bed.

'Hello, beautiful!' he said, his eyes smiling, and then he went on his way. Just two words, but they were enough. Always highly susceptible to any form of flattery, I responded immediately by returning his smile as he went back down the ward.

I never saw him again. It wasn't necessary. He had given back to me my ego. . . . I was a healthy young woman who just happened to have arthritis, that was all. They had put me in that particular ward because there happened to be a bed vacant, and quite honestly, I don't think they quite knew what to do with me.

I lay back and closed my eyes, and treated myself to a delightful scene where I skipped through a meadow with Frank and the girls trying to keep up with me. The meadow was bright with buttercups, and the handles of the skipping-ropes were scarlet, with little silver bells which tinkled as I skipped along. . . .

# 4

No experience, so they say, is ever wasted, and during the five weeks I lay resting myself so thoroughly I'd have made Rip Van Winkle appear to have St Vitus's Dance, I learnt two indisputable truths: one being that the nurses are underpaid angels and overworked slaves; and the other being that baked beans are very, very good for you.

When my daughters, now with children of their own, complain bitterly to me that good shin of beef and vitamin-packed boiled eggs are fiercely rejected in favour of baked beans, I can dismiss their anxiety with a knowledgeable smile. I was, the hospital told me, on a high protein diet; protein deficiency was then thought to be a contributory factor to rheumatoid arthritis, and baked beans appeared on my tray at every single meal.

Breakfast bacon, lunch-time stew, supper-time boiled fish, all arrived flanked by a huge mound of baked beans in tomato sauce.

Is it any wonder that now, all these years later, I shudder at the very sight of a tin, averting my eyes when I walk past that particular shelf in the supermarket.

As my particular treatment consisted of complete and utter rest, I wasn't, in spite of impassioned pleading, allowed to walk to the bathroom. When I became constipated, and hadn't 'been' for ten whole days, I explained, as nicely as I could, that the mere sight of a bed-pan was enough to paralyse my intestines, but they refused to listen.

The sister in charge of that ward, a tall, gaunt woman

with eyes that could have been taken out and replaced with glass marbles, so expressionless were they, told me I was being stubborn, and threatened me with enemas and worse. I told her I was honestly trying to co-operate.

'I know we're all made the same, and I know all about mock modesty,' I explained, trying desperately to make her understand. 'It's just that the thought of someone else having to walk to the sluice with the fruits of my endeavour makes me feel ashamed and humiliated, and *diminished*. It's a kind of mental block.'

But the kind of block sister was interested in wasn't a mental one. She pursed her thin lips until they almost disappeared.

'Patients who make an issue out of their natural functions are a menace to the smooth running of the ward, Mrs Joseph. You'll be dosed when the drugs trolley comes round this evening, and then if you insist on taking this obstinate attitude, we'll have to resort to other means.'

She said OTHER MEANS in capital letters, then took a step nearer to my bed, and I shrank back against my pillows.

'Patients with arthritis must have a complete bowel evacuation every single day. The intestines are teeming with bacteria, you know.'

She walked away on her quarter-to-three feet, her crêpe soles slapping away on the polished floor, and I closed my eyes and whiled away the next hour worrying about being constipated, and having every one of my tissues teeming with bacteria.

I remembered what I'd read in the latest book I'd read on my complaint:

'Your bowel elimination is slow because you cannot have enough exercise, then you start taking laxatives, which upset the tone of your intestinal tract. You eat little and become under-nourished and subject to digestive upsets. You move around in a vicious circle, of sluggishness, worry, anxiety, and all the conditions that favour arthritis.'

I remembered that water had been suggested as a cure, so I raised myself up and drank a glass of the tepid, acrid-smelling liquid on my locker, then lay down again and worried some more.

The necessity of using bed-pans didn't worry Bright Eyes on my left at all. She would gaily shame the whole ward by demanding one smack in the middle of visiting time, and once I'd been embarrassed almost to the point of hysteria by the sound of her passing wind and tearing toilet paper behind her screen just as the enrolling member of the Mothers' Union was telling me they were praying for me.

By the end of the fourth week, no fewer than eight of the patients had died, the old lady on my right who had called in vain for her niece Doris being the first to go. The procedure was always the same.

First there was a change in the victim's breathing pattern. It became hoarse and more laboured, then, as if ordered to, the entire ward became silent.

A deathly hush I'd call it, if I was trying to be face-tious . . . .

When it was all over, two nurses, usually the most junior, would disappear behind the flower-printed screens round the bed, and the laying-out process would take place.

'That new place in town, you know, the Emporium, I went dancing there last night,' I heard one little nurse tell her helpmate, as they did unspeakable things to the newly passed-on patient on my right.

'Many partners?'

'Lift her up a bit, that's right.'

'I laddered a stocking on the way there . . . . No, turn her over again, I want to pull the draw-sheet out my side. . . . And it rained, and I hadn't got a headscarf with me, and you know how frizzy my hair goes in the rain, then I stopped right opposite this bloke in the Paul Jones. Thought he was a right comic, he did. Danced

46

with me for the rest of the evening, but didn't bring me home when I told him where the Nurses' Home was. He called me Florence.'

'She doesn't look bad now, does she? Pass her comb over, and I'll tidy her hair up a bit. Why Florence?'

'Nightingale, dope.'

That first time, I was horrified. Where was their respect for the dead? The deference surely due to a still-warm corpse?

Then I realized this was the only way they could do what they had to do, by remaining completely uninvolved, or at least trying to. I ended up by marvelling at their courage.

Down each side of the ward, behind the beds, were four double french windows leading out on to a stone terrace, a covered one, the kind monks walk along chanting psalms. It was through these doors the newly departed and freshly laid-out were wheeled.

It was all done so discreetly that I don't remember ever actually seeing one go. Their mattresses were left out in the air for a while, and the next day the bed would be filled with yet another old lady, her grey hair fanning out on the pillow, her gnarled hands folded over her quivering chest.

Frank came to see me on the evenings he could get a baby-sitter for the children. Marilyn, he told me, had lost a front tooth, and had made a big dramatic scene, accusing him of laughing at her, and refusing to go to school. She had taken to talking with her mouth clamped tight shut. Katy had told her that she looked like a witch, evoking more floods of tears, and Mrs Barlowe had reported that our younger daughter had stirred half a pound of brussels sprouts round in the lavatory pan, and sworn on her very life that she'd seen a fairy fly through the window and do it.

'It's because she's missing me,' I said. 'Behaving badly is just her little way of expressing her insecurity.'

Frank laughed. 'But Katy's always had a penchant for

stirring things round the lavatory pan. It's one of her endearing quirks, love. Remember your pearl earrings, and my Christmas cigar?'

A strict rule of the hospital was that children under the age of eight were not allowed to visit. I would have protested about it, but didn't want my two sensitive little girls (does every mother think her children are a-quiver with sensitivity?) to see the old ladies gasping out their last breath in the rows of beds. Now, looking back, I can see that they would have been merely fascinated, but a mother has to be a grandmother before she can accept a truth like that.

When my small grandson Jamie visited me recently as I lay in bed after an operation to restore a knee joint, he was obviously disappointed to see *two* feet sticking out from beneath my cage. He had been sure, Katy told me, that they had cut off my leg!

At the end of the fourth week, the consultant rheumatologist came and stood by my bed, and told me that they had decided I ought to go into a hospital sixty miles away, a place where I would have specialized treatment.

He was very busy, obviously tired, and only trying to help, but at first I refused to listen, even when he told me how lucky I was to have got a place. He had written to the medical director himself, enlarging on my case, he told me, and he made it sound as if the waiting-list was at least five years long, and that if I didn't go I might just as well resign myself to a wheelchair.

'You have the virulent form of a progressive disease,' he said, 'and there you'll have peat baths, and exercises, and although they can't promise a cure, I know they can arrest the development of your symptoms.'

He sat down on the edge of my bed, and Sister, hovering the correct three paces behind him, looked so shocked, I wondered if the neck-line of my nightie was too low, and instinctively placed one hand over my bosom.

I assured him that my gratitude knew no bounds, but

that I couldn't possibly go; that I'd been away from my family long enough as it was, that I was so rested that I wouldn't need to sleep for at least six months. I told him I was sure my children were developing anxiety symptoms.

'They *need* me,' I went on. 'I'll worry about them so much, the treatment won't do me any good.'

I told him I felt marvellous, that I hadn't had so much as a twinge for three whole days, and that I would get up there and then and run down the ward, just to prove it.

He sat there and heard me out, whilst Sister raised her gimlet eyes ceilingwards, as if praying for patience to tide her over to my next remark.

'How long would I have to stay there, just supposing I went?' I asked at last, and he smiled.

'Only for about two months. The average length of stay is three months, but you've had your bed-rest here. Now they can concentrate on the treatment, and getting you mobile again. Talk it over with your husband when he comes in this evening. I'll be around, so I'll have a word with him first.'

He patted my shoulder and walked away, his white coat flying open, the matter quite settled in his own mind, I knew, and Sister came back and talked to me about ungrateful patients, and said the graveyards were full of indispensable people, and some patients didn't know when they were well off.

'I *know* I'm well off. I just want to go home,' I told her, and she softened suddenly and said that the children could come up and peep at me through the window at the weekend, if I liked.

The thought of their two little noses pressed up against the glass upset me so much I couldn't swallow my baked beans at supper-time, and I wasn't surprised to find, when Frank came in at visiting time that the doctor had already talked to him, and convinced him that we really had no choice.

'They're going to let you home for a weekend before

49

you go away again, and they'll lay on a car to take you all the way there. They don't think you're well enough to go by train.'

He sat there, looking worried, and I hated myself for being the cause of all his worry, and not for the first time I wished I were the type who could cry easily. I've always envied women who can let a stray tear slide slowly down their cheeks at a crucial moment, but it was useless, even though I concentrated fiercely on a mental image of myself growing old and crippled, being passed from one institution to another, the girls growing up without knowing me, and Frank replacing me with someone loose-limbed . . . .

'What is another eight weeks out of our lives?' he was saying. 'Mother has offered anyway to take the girls for two weeks to give Mrs Barlowe a break. I can take them down by train on Sunday, and be back in time to see you off.'

His parents had moved to Middlesex, and lived in a house with a little stream winding slowly through the front garden, a high hedge of honeysuckle at the back, and a swing hanging from the thick twisted branches of an old apple tree. The girls would be happy there, I knew.

'That would give me just one day with them,' I said slowly, and reached for Frank's hand. 'Can't you see I can't go away from them again? If I see them I'll never be able to leave them. Don't you see?'

'Then I'll take them before you come home,' said Frank, ever practical, and he made me laugh as usual, and as we laughed I knew we had no choice, and that he was right. I would see them and explain that I had to go away again, and just hope they were old enough to understand. If I refused I might never get the opportunity again, and it was for their sakes I had to go.

For the rest of that week I was allowed to get up for a little longer each day, to walk to the bathroom on legs that wobbled, and to sit in a chair by the side of my bed, writing letters and reading books from the mobile library that was wheeled round by jolly ladies wearing mauve overalls and jolly smiles, voluntary members of the hospital's Friendly Society.

I even got out my knitting, only to be caught at it by the rheumatologist, who almost snatched it from me in horror. Apparently my idea of 'keeping my fingers going' by knitting was quite wrong.

'The position of holding your arms close to your sides as you knit is very harmful,' he told me. 'Crochet work would be better if you feel you must be doing something, but knitting is one of the most harmful occupations for anyone with arthritis. And never sit with your legs crossed, or your ankles,' he added for good measure, and so I sat there on my uncomfortable little hard chair, feet obediently side by side, hands idle in my lap, and wished and willed the hours away.

As I had predicted, the state of my bowels reverted to normal, and I wallowed in a hot bath each morning, feeling really clean for the first time in weeks.

I was still losing weight, in spite of the high protein diet. The first time I got dressed, my suspender belt dangled round my hips, making my stockings wrinkle in unglamorous folds round my ankles. Staff Nurse told me kindly that my loss of weight meant that my muscles were wasting and losing substance, and Bright Eyes told me that I looked as if I'd been 'spoke-shaved', a Lancashire expression I'd never heard before, which fascinated me.

By 5.45 on the Saturday morning I was all packed and ready to go, trembling a little with the exertion, sitting by my bed and glancing at my watch every three minutes or so, astonished to find that at least half an hour hadn't passed since the last time I looked at it. I was to be taken home in the out-patients' ambulance, a vehicle designed something like a tumbril, with seats either side and let-down steps at the back.

When the driver, a gaunt young man with a white face

and protruding eyes who looked as if something un-speakable had happened to him in the woodshed in his youth, finally came into the ward at around 9.30, I was so glad to see him, I almost threw myself into his arms.

I said goodbye to Bright Eyes, who surprised me by kissing me soundly, and telling me that she would miss me, and making me promise to 'have faith', and as I walked down the ward, all the little old ladies who were conscious raised white heads from their pillows and waved feebly. I told myself I would never forget them, a promise more readily made than kept, and as I went past Sister's little office, she looked up from telephoning, and actually smiled at me.

Saying goodbye to anyone, under any circumstances, always has the power to demoralize me. I once astonished a milkman who was leaving to take up another round by being so overcome I couldn't even wish him luck. I often think that he must have been sure that I'd been nursing a secret passion for him, and regretting that fact that he hadn't made a pass at me over the milk bottles . . . .

And so with my throat choked with the tears I couldn't shed, I followed the driver of the ambulance out into the forecourt. He turned and grinned at me:

'You can sit up alongside me, love, if you like,' he said, and as we drove out of the hospital gates, I gazed enraptured through the windscreen, going into a mild form of ecstasy over the dear little houses, the green lawns, the rose bushes, the healthy people walking their dogs, the healthy people carrying loaded shopping bags. Even a dirty old tramp spitting in the gutter looked endearing to me.

I told the driver how long I'd been in hospital, why I'd been in hospital, all about my treatment, how old I was, the names of my two little girls, what Frank did for a living; we got stuck in a traffic jam as we drove through the town, and I told him which school I'd attended, what style I was going to wear my hair when I managed to get to a hairdresser, and when he turned the ambulance into our familiar crescent of houses, and I saw Marilyn and Katy swinging on the gate, I told him, my voice choked with emotion, that in everyone's life there came moments of happiness so exquisite that it was all too much to bear, and didn't he agree?

He turned his dazed, bulbous, pale blue eyes full on me.

'If you say so, love,' he said, and I realized that was the first time I'd given him a chance to say a single word.

Frank must have been watching from the window, because he came down the path, a tea-towel in his hand, thanked him and pressed a ten shilling note into his hand, as I walked over to the children.

Their *faces* were bigger, that was my first reaction. In five weeks they had grown, and if I'd imagined them hurling themselves into my outstretched arms, with cries of 'Mummy, Mummy, you're home!' I would have been disappointed. But this was life, not fiction, and besides I knew them too well.

Katy hung her head, put her thumb in her mouth, and looked as if she were going to burst into tears, and Marilyn said, 'I'm the best in my class at reading, and Katy's pulled another piece of paper off her wall, and drunk half a bottle of cough medicine, and we made some fudge, and it stuck to the pan, and Daddy put the pan in the dustbin because he couldn't get it off . . . .'

'That's marvellous, and never mind,' I said, and we all went into the house, and it was as though all the colours had suddenly become sharpened and more vivid. The browns and reds of the little square carpet in the living room glowed, and the rather grubby upholstery of the two utility fireside chairs gleamed as it if were gold brocade, and although the day was warm, Frank had lit a fire in the grate, and the copper coal-scuttle shone with pin-points of light.

It was the most beautiful room in the whole world, worth nothing less than a three-page spread in *Homes and Gardens* – and that is the reaction I've always had whenever I've come back from hospital.

The *softness* of everything, the cosiness, the tidiness –
everyone who has looked after my home when I've had
to go away always seems to be cast in a tidier mould than
me . . . .

I sat down by the fire, and Katy came and climbed
rather shyly on to my knee, burying her head under my
chin. Not to be outdone, Marilyn, six years old, and built
like an overlarge seven, climbed on to the other knee,
and I saw that Katy's blue jumper was on inside out, and
that Marilyn was wearing odd socks, and already the old
ladies in the hospital ward seemed a hundred light years
away . . . .

# 5

I couldn't bear to think that the very next day I was to be parted from the children again, but there it was, and if you can't alter things then you just learn to live with them, as my aunt was always saying.

The girls were still sitting on my knees, one of which was protesting violently, when Frank brought me a cup of coffee, the first I'd had since going into hospital, and it tasted like nectar straight from the gods.

Marilyn told me all about her new friend Pat, who had recently come to live in the Crescent.

'She's six weeks older than me, but she's bigger than me,' she confided.

'Is she *really*?' I marvelled, and Frank told me that it was quite true, and we marvelled together. A knock sounded at the back door, and best friend Pat came in; Marilyn made her stand back-to-back with her, and there *was* a good half-inch difference in their heights.

Pat stared hard at me for a full five minutes, and then told me that the cat next door to them had had three kittens.

'Giblets,' she said solemnly, and arms round each other, the girls went off to see. Frank told me we were having fish and chips from the shop in the village for lunch, then the milk lady called for the weekly money, and told me how thin I was, and when I told her I was going away to another hospital, said she hoped they weren't going to use me for a guinea-pig.

'That's what they do,' she said, putting the money away in the leather purse she carried round her waist.

'They *experiment*.' She went on to tell me about a new drug for arthritis which changed women into men, making them grow hair on their faces, and develop voices as deep as Paul Robeson's.

The horse which pulled the milk float was getting restless. We could hear it making whinnying noises, but the milk lady was well into her stride. She'd had arthritis, she said; been bent almost double with it, but she'd got these little pills from the herbalist in the village, and how she'd sweated! No one had ever sweated like she'd sweated. Even the mattress had been wringing wet, it had poured from her like a river, but after a week of going around with permanent globules of perspiration on her face, and rotting her stockings and the insides of her shoes, she'd been cured. And if I could find a piece of paper she'd write the name of the tablets down for me, and it was really nice to see me back, even looking so thin and poorly.

When she'd gone Katy came and climbed back on to my knee. I stared into the fire, and when Frank asked me what I was thinking about, I told him I was trying to decide whether having hairs on my face and a voice like Paul Robeson's wouldn't be preferable to paddling around in a pool of my own sweat.

Katy seemed to have dropped off to sleep, and shifting her weight on to my good knee, I felt her forehead.

'She's a bit hot,' I said, and Frank admitted that she hadn't slept all that well the night before.

'I expect it's the excitement of you coming home. She feels things much too deeply for her age. Here, let me have her. I'll take her up to bed, and a good sleep will put her right.'

I followed him upstairs, my legs aching with the effort, and we tucked Katy into bed with her carpet sweeper, an article she'd insisted on sleeping with ever since she'd been given it as a birthday present. She wound the tatty ribbon of her precious suck-a-blanket round her thumb, smiled at us, and was asleep again in minutes.

Trying to make as little noise as possible, I took the case containing their summer dresses out of the wardrobe, and told Frank I was going to spend all afternoon letting down the hems.

'It's bound to be much warmer down in Middlesex,' I said, and Frank, like a true Lancastrian, denied it hotly, saying that was a myth, and anyway I hadn't come home to start sewing straight away.

'Wouldn't be surprised if a few friends don't drop in this evening,' he said. 'Muriel and Derek, and Harold (his brother) and Marjorie. They said they would, but they won't stay long, they know we want to be on our own.'

'Do we?' I asked, and out on the wide landing, he put his arm around me, and I leaned against him, and his sweater had that smell of tobacco and gear-oil I was so familiar with, and I kissed him, and he said it was time he went down to the village for the fish and chips, and I said was it any wonder I loved him so much when he was so romantic?

Being a seasoned southerner now of twenty years' standing, I don't know how it is up there in the north of England, but in those days, friends really did just 'drop in'. There was no telephoning first to see it if was convenient; for one thing, hardly any of our friends at that time could afford a telephone. They just took it for granted that they were welcome at any time, and that evening, after we'd put the girls to bed, no fewer than six couples were gathered together in the living-room, all come to say hello and goodbye, and wish me well.

The men congregated at one side of the room, and the women at the other, the former to talk about football and cars, and the women about far more important things.

Women's Lib hadn't been thought of then. We saw nothing in the least unusual that we were excluded from the men's conversation, and the summer dresses were passed round, and hems turned down, to the accompani-

57

ment of the day's cricket scores on the radio.

I didn't talk about the hospital I'd been in for the past five weeks, or about the one I was going to. Muriel said she would come round the next morning and give me a home perm, and each friend made outrageous claims about the solace they had been offering Frank whilst I'd been away. It was all good, clean fun, and we laughed so much that my next-door neighbour rapped on the wall.

Were we really so innocent in those days, or was it merely that no one had invented the terms permissive society, or wife-swapping?

Around nine o'clock – the time the ward lights would have been lowered, and the old ladies fallen into their uneasy slumbers – the room was thick with cigarette smoke, beer was being drunk out of cups as we'd run out of glasses, and the 'boys' had been out twice to Annie's, the selling-out shop on the corner, for reinforcements.

I was so tired, my eyelids kept drooping, and I could see Frank watching me with anxiety in his eyes. I thought of all the evenings he must have sat alone in that room, with just the radio and his textbooks for company, and I forced myself to try to stay awake, but when at last we were alone, I admitted that I might be just a little tired, and we went upstairs, leaving the debris to be dealt with in the morning.

After the hard hospital bed, our double mattress felt as if it was floating on air, and I hardly remembered my head touching the pillow. The first thing I knew was when I opened my eyes, and saw Marilyn standing by the bed.

'Katy's making a funny noise,' she said, and I got up and went through into their room, grasping at the furniture as I went to help me walk. Katy was fast asleep with her mouth open, and beads of perspiration on her rounded forehead.

I touched her; she was blessedly cool, and she woke and sat straight up in bed, making the transition from sleep to wakefulness the way only a child can do.

'Is it today we go to London on the train, Mummy?' she asked, and I put my arms round her, and told her that indeed it was, and that Grannie had written to say they'd had the swing mended, and that if they were good they could go into town one day to the zoo in Regent's Park.

'And see the monkeys? The ones with red bottoms?'

'The very ones,' I promised, and Katy said she liked going on a train.

'Why can't you come with us?' she asked.

I explained as carefully as I could that I had to go away again, but that soon I'd be home, and then I'd never go away again. As I talked I was thinking how frail she looked, with her little pansy face, and her long soft brown hair and eyes, and my heart sank at the prospect of leaving them all again.

I realized again how ultra-sensitive she was, and remembered reading that a child's mind could be permanently damaged by being separated from her mother, at just Katy's tender age. I saw her growing up inhibited, unable to mix with other children, a loner, ostracized by children who haven't suffered the traumatic experience of having their mother returned to them, only to be taken away from her in the space of twenty-four hours . . . .

'Is it time to go now, Mummy?' Katy asked me suddenly, her brown eyes sparkling with anticipation. 'Going on a train, and going to the zoo are my two very favourite things. . . .'

An affluent friend with a car was running Frank and the girls to the station, and I waved them off from the door, Frank weighted down with the big case containing the newly let-down summer dresses, and Marilyn and Katy bouncing down the path by his side, being reminded to turn and wave to me as they climbed into the back of the car.

I went slowly upstairs, and started to pack my own case – nighties, dressing-gown, face flannels, talcum powder – tearless as usual, but with a heavy feeling round my heart as if I'd eaten a whole uncooked Christmas pudding. I went round the house, tidying drawers, checking the pantry for ready-cooked foods for Frank's two weeks alone, and baked two apple pies, an effort that left me exhausted, so that the five minutes I'd planned on sleeping on my bed turned into two hours, and I awoke stiff and cold, with my ankles feeling as if they were turning the wrong way, and my knees burning with the familiar grinding ache.

Frank came home around midnight, and we stayed awake talking till two o'clock and told each other that eight weeks was a mere nothing, and that I'd be home again before either of us could say Jack Knife.

'But we never say Jack Knife,' I said, and Frank laughed, and said that was the spirit, and that he knew my sense of humour would see me through. I insisted on getting up with him the next morning, and cooking bacon and eggs for his breakfast, feeling it was the last proper meal he'd have until I came back.

And at 10.30 the official car came to pick me up.

It was large and black, like a funeral hearse. The driver wore a peaked cap, a navy-blue suit shiny from too much sitting behind the wheel, and an expression that said clearly he'd been told I was a terminal case, and must be treated with reverent concern.

I could see that he was plainly disappointed when I opened the door to him, obviously capable of walking down the path all by myself.

My next-door neighbour waved goodbye to me from her porch, and I waved back and smiled, then the milk float turned into the Crescent, and I reminded the milk lady that one pint would be enough until the children came back from London.

She clearly didn't hold with me going into hospital again, and before she could start telling me about the sweat-inducing tablets once more, I got into the car.

'I'll sit here in the front with you, if you don't mind,' I

told the driver, scorning the tartan blanket neatly folded on the back seat, and he said he thought I'd have wanted to put my legs up, and I said that where I was going there'd be plenty of time for that.

As he started the car, I took a last look at the house, with its green lawn, and long border of sweet alyssum and blue lobelia. A watery sun was beginning to peep out from behind high-banked cloud, and the driver said it didn't look as if we were going to have any summer that year. For the first few miles, he ran through a resumé of the past seven summers, and expounded his theory that we were quickly running into another Ice Age.

'Well, I won't be around to see it,' I said, and he glanced sideways at me, and I wondered again just what he thought was wrong with me.

'I've got arthritis, that's all,' I told him, and he couldn't have been more gratified if I'd said I'd got advanced leprosy or some obscure but fatal type of gut rot.

'Terrible thing,' he said, neatly skirting a roundabout. 'Scourge of the nation. More man-hours lost by arthritis than any other complaint, and you're so young, aren't you? Bad enough when you get it when you're old enough to expect it, anyway. There's not much they can do for it once it's taken hold, is there?'

'Children can get it,' I said, and remembered reading that it could be inherited. I saw in my mind's eye Marilyn and Katy in a wheelchair apiece, their lovely straight young limbs twisted and distorted, and me blaming myself for ever having them, and bringing them into a world where they would live out their lives in pain and suffering.

'Are you going to die?' Marilyn had asked me once with great interest over her bowl of breakfast cereal. 'Laura Jamieson's father died, and she told me he was in a box in their front room. She said I could go and look at him on my way home from school if I wanted to.'

61

'I won't like it if you die,' said Katy, her brown eyes brimming, staring at me through a milk moustache, and I assured them both that I had no intention of dying, that I would soon be back home again, and that I was going to be looked after by a lot of kind nurses and doctors, who would make me walk properly again. I reminded them that this time, definitely, we would all skip together on the lawn.

The driver was telling me about a friend of his who'd been cured by having bees sting him all over his naked body, and who had changed from a hopeless cripple into a man who ran two miles each morning before breakfast, and who had taken up rugger once again at the age of fifty-three.

The watery sun had by now completely disappeared, and he had switched on the windscreen wipers to cope with the increasing drizzle. The car was so well fitted-up that I had a pair all to myself, and found I was unable to stop my eyes from swinging from side to side, following their rhythm.

He was a very good driver, gliding up to traffic-lights and using the gears with smooth dexterity, and I tried to feel grateful that I was getting all this for free. I told myself that I was indeed privileged, that I was being given V.I.P. treatment, and that all over the country were crippled, house-bound women who would give their all to have the chance of a place in the specialized unit over the other side of the Pennines.

I beckoned wildly to my mental Pollyanna; I tried to be *glad* that I was going, but I couldn't help thinking how uncomplicated a session of bee stings would have been compared to my way of setting out in search of relief.

The driver started to hum underneath his breath, and as he was apparently tone-deaf it took me a while to fathom the tune. It turned out to be a syncopated version of Abide With Me, and cheered me up no end . . . .

'Nearly there,' he said, after almost three hours' driving, and we turned into a long road bordered with rhododendron bushes, their dark green leaves shiny and almost black with rain. The hospital was at the foot of the hill, on the right, and it might have been the residence of some wealthy gentleman, if there had been cars instead of white ambulances parked in the drive.

'Looks like a prison, doesn't it?' my driver remarked as he got my case out of the boot. As we went up the steps into the wide dark entrance hall, and the big glass doors swung to behind us, I told him that if only I'd had T.B. they might have sent me to Switzerland where I could have lain all day on a balcony and watched the sun sparkling on the mountains.

'They don't do that now. They can cure T.B. with injections,' my driver explained kindly, putting my case down, and bidding me a sad farewell.

There was no one in sight. The reception desk was deserted; it was dark and gloomy, and even the silence smelt damp. I looked for a bell to ring, found nothing, and stood there, shifting my weight from one foot to the other, and wondering if everyone had gone home.

I wanted to go home too, and was thinking how marvellous it would be if they'd closed the whole place down because of some unknown virus, when a porter appeared from nowhere, as if someone had rubbed on a lamp and summoned him up. His appearance added to the illusion.

He was a gnome-like tiny man, and I warmed to him on sight, because he smiled at me, a gash of a smile, stretching from one pointed ear to the other. He told me to 'sit me down', and he would ring for a nurse to come. Smiling back at him, I walked obediently over to a bench by the window, and 'sat me down'.

I'm quite prepared to admit that we can't go around with inane grins on our faces, but oh, what a difference a smile can make at the right moment.

I stopped thinking about pain and suffering, and my two little girls over two hundred miles away, and Frank starting another session of coming home to a wifeless house, boiling himself an egg in a pan that hadn't been washed for seven weeks. The little porter put the telephone down still smiling at me, and I went on smiling back, and soon a nursing orderly in a white coat with a face to match came towards me and, picking up my case, told me to follow her.

We walked along a corridor and into a large room lined with rows of old ladies in wheelchairs, their hands lying idle and twisted in their laps, watching what could laughingly be called a group of patients doing exercises.

These were fully dressed, and the physiotherapist in the middle, a middle-aged lady with black hair skewered on top of her head cottage-loaf style, was urging them to raise their arms.

'Arms up!' she called, lifting her voice on the 'up', and I saw that more arms stayed down than went up. I asked the orderly carrying my case if only the worst cases of arthritis were sent to that particular hospital. She turned round, and said that was indeed the case but I wasn't to worry, because they worked wonders, and she'd seen patients come in bent like corkscrews, and then after treatment, go out with the springing step of a ballet dancer.

Looking back over my shoulder at the group of gymnasts, now trying in vain to clasp their hands behind their backs, I found this difficult to believe. But it was nice to hear all the same, and I followed my optimistic orderly up a wide flight of stairs, one step at a time, slowly and painfully, seeing myself in eight weeks' time running on the tips of my toes, arms outstretched à la Fonteyn, across the wide wide forecourt into the astonished arms of Frank and the children, who waited for me in the shelter of the dripping rhododendron bushes . . . .

# 6

Going into an unknown hospital for an unspecified length of time is a bit like starting to serve a prison sentence, but worse, because you have the feeling that you haven't done anything to deserve it . . . .

There were four beds in my little ward, two of which were empty, but the one next to mine was occupied by a stick-thin middle-aged woman, introduced to me by the nursing orderly as Miss Evans.

She was so thin she would have made Twiggy look like the fat lady at a circus. She smiled at me, a sweet, uncomplaining smile, and told me that she'd been in bed for twelve weeks, and was perfectly happy to stay there for another twelve, as she lived with her married sister and her family, and knew that she was a BURDEN.

I've always thought that being a burden was bad enough, but to *admit* to being one is even worse, and I knew instinctively that Miss Evans was the sort of woman who enjoyed having bad health, and my heart sank at the prospect of living in such close proximity to her for the next two months.

I wasn't exactly laughing my head off, either. I don't wake up properly until noon, and then it's time for my afternoon sleep. I used to think this meant that I was niggly, until I read that the cause of my morning lethargy was my blood sugar not rising quickly enough . . . Miss Evans didn't look as if she even *had* any blood sugar!

The orderly showed me the cupboard where I had to hang my clothes.

'Come straight down to Surgery, dear. Miss Evans will

65

tell you where it is. I should give you a bath by right, but there just isn't time.'

I assured her that I had had my bath that morning, and that I could bath myself, thank you, and she said that too much of the independent spirit could be a detriment to getting well.

'With our complaint, we have to learn to accept help gracefully,' she said, and I wondered nastily why she said 'we' when she hadn't got arthritis. Miss Evans smiled sadly and told me that her sister did *everything* for her, and in my rebellious mood I mentally pitied the sister, and not poor Miss Evans – although now that I'm older, and have mellowed quite a lot, I can see that sympathy and pity were the two things that Miss Evans would have appreciated more than any other.

Undressing in front of a woman I'd only just met, without the benefit of a screen, made me embarrassed and I fumbled more than usual with fingers too swollen to do my bidding. I have a marvellous gadget for undoing zips, one of the few gadgets I have ever allowed myself, and even that turned awkward on me. It is a hook attached to a long cord, and the idea is that you hook it into the 'eye' of the zip, throw the cord over your shoulder, then pull the cord, so that the zip slides up, or down, as the case might be.

I couldn't, even if I'd wanted to, ask Miss Evans for help. Her hands and wrists were encased in white plaster, and I saw that her fingers sloped at an angle of almost ninety degrees. Leaning against her locker were a couple of plaster casts for her legs, great ugly monstrosities, with 'flipper' attachments, to keep her ankles from dropping as she slept.

She saw me looking at them, and told me that they were very uncomfortable, and that lying flat on her back in them meant she had no sleep at all, that she never closed her eyes most nights, but just lay there in agony, praying for the dawn.

'You'll be seeing the doctor now, dear,' she told me

kindly, 'and the first thing he'll do is put you to bed for a month. That's the treatment here, unless of course your case is as far gone as mine – bed-rest for four weeks, then treatment for at least another four'. She sighed, and it seemed happily. 'Of course they can't do anything for me. Mine came on in the "change", and that's the worst kind. My hormones are completely hay-wire. I've been in a wheelchair for four years, and my legs are bent right up. They say they've never seen knees like mine. I've been having them drained once a month, and each time they get a whole bowl of fluid from them. Yellow. But it always comes back again. They'll never straighten them now, but I suppose they feel they must try.'

I shuddered; got the better of my zip gadget, and slipped out of my dress.

'I've already had my bed-rest period in another hospital,' I told her, turning my back as I wriggled out of my bra by the simple expedient of swivelling it round to the front and unhooking it. 'I'm just here for the treatment. Peat baths, massage – that kind of thing.'

Although my back was to her, I could feel her nod, and knew that the nod was conveying gently that nothing they did would do me the slightest good.

'If you are seeing the doctor, *he* won't take any notice when you tell him you've already been to bed for your complete rest, dear,' her gentle voice assured me. 'He doesn't like other doctors interfering with what he thinks is best. There's a young lady in the next room about your age, and he put her to bed for nine weeks. He's like that, stubborn, and I must say it would be nice company for me if we were up here together all day long. I do get lonely, not that I complain. I'm never depressed you see because I have FAITH. There's nothing like FAITH for keeping you smiling through your tears, and that's what I've always done, smiled through mine.'

Poor, dear Miss Evans. Now, looking back, I can see how lonely she was, and that her illness was *important* to her, but then, over twenty years ago, I was young, impatient with mine, wanting above all else not to dwell on it; wanting to ignore it as much as possible, and just get on with living.

I'd made up my mind that doctor or no doctor, they weren't going to put me to bed again. Already the place had got under my skin, and Miss Evans's passive acceptance of her arthritis made me want to scream out loud. Pollyanna, I decided, had left me at the door, and was lurking outside somewhere amongst all those dank and dripping rhododendron bushes . . . .

On my way down to the surgery, I passed women walking on crutches, women walking with sticks, grey-faced and worn. And paying a quick call to the bathroom, I saw with horror that three of the lavatories were without doors, wide of frontage, to allow for the easy entry of wheelchairs, and even the fourth door was without any form of lock or bolt.

In the little room adjoining the surgery, a harassed nurse told me I was late, weighed me hurriedly, and told me I was over a stone underweight for my height and age. She said it as if I'd deliberately lost the stone on my way there, and when I said that I couldn't understand it as I'd lived exclusively on baked beans and sago pudding for the past five weeks, not to mention whole mountain ranges of mashed potatoes, she made no reply, merely glanced at me with an invisible sign on her furrowed forehead, which said PATIENTS ARE NOT ALLOWED TO MAKE JOKES HERE!

It was almost lunch-time, and the doctor was obviously in a hurry.

'Which joints trouble you the most?' he asked, and almost falling over myself with the effort of trying to be lucid and helpful, I told him my hands, wrists, shoulders, knees, ankles, big toes, the back of my neck, and that sometimes my bottom hurt when I sat down.

He laid his pencil down wearily, and massaged a spot in between his bushy eyebrows, so quickly I modified my list to two places, my hands and knees, and he wrote this down on a notepad, then asked me the next question:

'Which troubles you the most, the pain or the deformity?'

I tried to think. I sat there, trying to be helpful. I wanted to impress him with my intelligence and willingness to co-operate, but I honestly didn't *know* the answer. And the more I tried to be honest, the more my thoughts wandered, and I found myself thinking about the girls, wondering if they were happy down in London; had Katy been sickening for something before they left, or was she at that very moment running about in the lovely garden with its swing and high hedge of honeysuckle?

Surely it wouldn't be raining quite so hard down there? I tried to remember if I'd packed their wellingtons, and knew I hadn't, seeing them standing there, forgotten, in the cupboard underneath the stairs . . . .

'The pain or the deformity?' asked the doctor again, and I said 'Both', which was quite obviously the wrong answer, as he raised his eyes ceilingwards, as if in prayer.

It wasn't a very satisfactory interview. I was doing my best to convince him that it was all a mistake that I'd been sent there in the first place; that compared to the patients I'd already seen, I was so mobile I could have been considered as a likely candidate for the next Olympics, and he, in his turn, was trying to impress on me the gravity of my complaint.

He wasn't to know that my only defence against it was, and always has been, a *flippancy* and a refusal to believe in its seriousness, but he did agree with me that I had already served my bed-rest period, and said I could start treatments straight away.

He told me I was to have a course of peat baths, under-water massage, ultra-violet ray sessions, because of my skinniness and general debility, exercises, plaster casts for my wrists, and soluble aspirin, taken three times a day.

I asked him why I wasn't to be given cortisone, or

ACTH (adrenocorticotropic hormone), being a mine of information on these new drugs on account of reading a book from the library, but the doctor shook his head.

'We'll try aspirin first,' he said firmly. 'I am accused at times of being old-fashioned, but I believe in trying something which has the minimum of side-effects.' He glanced at the letter from the hospital back home. 'Later we may put you on a course of gold injections, we have good results in some cases from gold.' Then he scribbled something down on his pad, tore off a leaf, and handed it to the nurse, standing silently by his desk.

I thanked him, and he took off his glasses, and smiled at me.

'You are young, and if you co-operate fully, I think I can promise you that your stay here will at least arrest your symptoms.'

'I've promised my children I'll be able to skip when I go home,' I told him, and he laughed, and the nurse ushered me out quickly before I gave any more indications that I could be human. Out in the tiny waiting-room, she wrote out a list of my treatments for the coming week and handed the form to me.

'Be on time for your appointments, otherwise you'll have to forgo your treatments,' she told me, and I promised faithfully, and went out into the wide corridor again.

And it was like being at school again, a new girl, on the first day of term; I stood there uncertainly, not knowing where to go, not knowing a soul apart from Miss Evans, lying still and uncomplaining in her little bed upstairs. Then I remembered I would have to go back upstairs to get dressed again, and I walked past all the wheelchairs ranged along the sides of the 'gymnasium', past all the shuffling hobbling ladies, all going I knew not where.

I walked as quickly as I could, trying hard not to limp, trying to convince myself, if nobody else, that I was there under false pretences, that I wasn't like them, and never would be. Never . . . .

Miss Evans was having her lunch, feeding herself awkwardly in her splints. I saw the struggle she had to lift the spoon to her mouth, and as I dressed there was a small voice screaming away inside me, telling me that I couldn't bear it, even if she could. That I'd rather be at home and a burden, amongst people who loved me, than there, in that dreadful place, swallowing aspirins, and wallowing in hot baths.

I could do all that at home, I told myself. I'd tell them that. I'd promise on my very life that I would lie all morning pickling myself in hot water, and that I would swallow aspirin tablets by the handful. If only they would let me OUT!

I'd forgotten to bring along my hand mirror, and as I tried to comb my too curly hair and add a layer of lipstick with the aid of the three-inch mirror from my handbag, a gong sounded from what seemed miles away.

'The food's very good,' Miss Evans told me, 'not that I have much of an appetite.' She was eagerly, albeit awkwardly, scraping her plate as she spoke, and I left her making a start on her pudding, thinking her beautiful negative thoughts, and went in search of the dining-room.

It was easy to find. All I had to do was to follow the straggling procession of women, some with walking frames, some on sticks, others on crutches, some being pushed along by orderlies, and just a few, like myself, getting there under their own limping steam.

I stood in the entrance of the dining-room, wondering where to sit.

Were all the places pre-arranged, or did one just sit anywhere? I felt as if all eyes were on me, and if I hadn't been hungry (arthritis has never affected my appetite) I'd have gone back upstairs and exchanged morbid pleasantries with Miss Evans.

Just then a girl around my own age spoke to me:

'You new here, honey?'

'New and petrified, and not feeling half so sweet as

71

honey,' I told her, and she grinned.

She had almost white-blonde hair, piled high, with dangling diamanté earrings and, bare-legged, was wearing a short summer dress in a bright orange shade. I liked her on sight.

'Come and sit with me,' she said. 'Come on. The two tables on the right are for patients on a diet. To be fat is a sin as far as arthritis is concerned.' She glanced at my navy-blue dress which fitted me like a sack, long before that style came into its own. 'Reckon you don't belong with them, honey.'

'Are you American?' I asked her, as we sat down at a long table, and she smiled and shook her head.

'Gee, no, honey. I'm as English as you, but I married a G.I. during the war, and I suppose his accent has kinda rubbed off on me.'

An orderly was setting down heaped-up plates of shepherd's pie in every place – huge mounds of fluffy toasted potatoes and a liberal helping of mince, flanked by the inevitable baked beans.

'I'm Sheila,' my new friend said, helping herself to tomato sauce and starting to eat with her fork held in her right hand, American style. I noticed that although her knuckles were swollen, and her fingers had the familiar sideways slope, her nails were painted a fierce pillar-box red, a shade at complete and utter variance with the colour of her dress.

'And I'm Marie,' I told her, and tried not to look at the table on our right, where orderlies standing behind the chairs were helping the patients to feed themselves, spooning the food into their mouths as if they were babies.

Sheila nudged me. 'Take no notice, honey. It does kinda bug you at first, but you're not going to be like that, neither am I. The old Doc here promised me that. Arthritis is like any other disease; you can have it mild, or you can have it bad, and we're young enough to benefit from the treatments. You on cortisone?'

'Soluble aspirins. How about you?'

'The same,' she told me. 'I've been here for four weeks now, and when I go home I'm reckoning on being fighting fit. I told the Doc, straight. "Just you concentrate on my hands and my feet, the rest of me is O.K. Just let me get back to my kids, that's all." '

All around me the plates of shepherd's pie, the best I'd ever tasted, were being demolished with such speed that I could see I was going to be left behind if I didn't stop talking. The woman on my right helped herself to her third dollop of tomato sauce, and I turned to Sheila.

'Is your husband coping with the children whilst you're away?'

She shook her head violently, putting the upswept pile of hair into instant jeopardy.

'What? That jerk? No, he went back to the States two years ago. Reckon he hadn't banked on having a sick wife to live with. My mum's looking after my two boys, and she's none too good herself, so the sooner I get back, the better.'

The plates were collected, and before the pudding came round (lavish helpings of jam sponge smothered in thick yellow custard), the medicine trolley was wheeled amongst the tables, lists were consulted, and the appropriate pills handed out.

'Food, tablets if you're on them, then food,' Sheila told me. 'That way it reduces stomach upsets. You'll be getting yours tomorrow, honey, when they've had time to sort you out.'

She started to eat her pudding. 'It may seem a bit disorganized the first day, but they know what they're doing. Have they told you what you're having this afternoon?'

I took my treatment slip from my handbag, and told her:

'Infra-red lamp, then under-water massage.'

She grinned. 'No need to look so worried, honey. There's an orderly down there in the treatment rooms

73

we call Big Annie. She's got muscles like Mr Universe, and she squirts water on your joints as you lie in a kind of shallow trough. The pressure's supposed to be terrific, but because you're lying submerged you don't feel it much, but first we have to lie on our beds for an hour and a half. You got good company in your room?'

I told her about Miss Evans, and she told me that she was in a ward of eight beds, five of them with patients on complete bed-rest, and that the nights were made hideous by groans and snores, interspersed by the odd scream.

I asked her about sleeping tablets, and she told me that they were frowned on by the doctors there, because a drugged sleep is a sleep where you lie in one position most of the time, and wake up stiffer than ever.

'I'm learning all the time,' I said, and she nodded.

'By the time you get out of here, honey, you'll be an *authority*, mark you me!'

Cups of hot, strong tea were brought round, and I told Sheila that my two little girls were down in London with their grannie.

'Let's get out of here and have a fag,' she said. 'We're allowed to smoke in the Lounge, and if we go now we'll just have time for one before resting time.'

I didn't smoke at that time, but I followed her gladly, and we sat down on a chintz-covered sofa, in front of an enormous coal fire. Sheila lit a cigarette, balanced it carefully between her lips, and from her cavernous handbag took out a roll of purple knitting.

'Keeps the fingers going,' she told me, and I hadn't the heart to contradict her, not just then. I leaned my head back against the chintz cover, and began to relax for the first time that day.

Staying in that hospital wasn't exactly going to be a picnic, but having Sheila for a friend was going to help to make it bearable.

'Where is everybody?' I asked her, staring round the huge and deserted lounge.

'Lying flat on their beds like good little girls,' said

74

Sheila, stopping knitting for long enough to blow a perfect smoke-ring up towards the high ceiling, before starting on another purple row . . . .

# 7

On my very first day in the specialist hospital it didn't take me long to find out that my new friend, Sheila, was of the opinion that rules were made to be broken.

'It's bed at half past nine,' she told me in disgust. 'A regular ten hours a night, that's what they say we must have. They teach us here the sort of life we're supposed to lead when we go back home, and that's a big laugh for a start.'

She was knitting in the lounge at a time when we were supposed to be lying flat on our beds for the after-lunch rest and, dropping a stitch, she said a word I'd only seen written on lavatory walls.

'I work full-time in a typing pool in Manchester, and I'd just like to see the expression on my supervisor's face if I told her I wanted to lie down for an hour after lunch. I rush and do my shopping in my lunch hour, pick up the kids from my mother's on the way home, and do my housework and washing and ironing when they're in bed. I can't *afford* to rest.'

'Doesn't your husband send you any money?' I asked her, stealing worried glances at the clock on the wall, not wanting to be caught disobeying the rules on my first day, and yet riveted to my chair by Sheila's forceful personality.

She went on knitting, using the thick steel needles as if they were battering rams.

'Disappeared,' she said. 'Done a bunk. I haven't had a penny from him since Christmas.'

'But that's awful,' I said, and she shifted the stub of

her cigarette from one corner of her mouth to the other.

'That's *life*, honey,' she said.

I told her I was going up to my room, and she looked disappointed in me, but didn't say anything, and I left her there, lighting another cigarette, a defiant, lonely figure in her orange frock, willing, I was sure, to do battle with the whole world if needs be. In my small ward, Miss Evans was lying obediently flat, her arms in their white plaster casts stretched out neatly by her side.

In the third bed, an enormously fat woman lay on her stomach, like a whale left stranded by the tide, her huge bottom encased in a short and hairy blue tweed skirt.

She opened one eye and winked at me.

'Hello, duck, I'm Myrtle,' she said, and Miss Evans said there was only twenty minutes of my lying-down time left, and if I was caught on my feet by one of the orderlies, I'd be sent to report to the doctor.

'And sent home?' I asked hopefully, and Myrtle laughed, a shaking belly laugh.

'Oh, it's not so bad once you get used to it. I've been here three months, and I come here in a wheelchair; now I'm walking on crutches.' She gave an almighty heave, and turned herself right way up. 'I'm supposed to lie on me stomach to help straighten me hips,' she explained. 'Hope you don't mind me bloomers drying on the radiator. You can send things to the laundry, but most of us do our own bits and pieces in the wash-basin. You get to know the times Sister comes round, and you can whip 'em off before she sees.'

She then told me that she'd had arthritis for ten years; that it had come on overnight after her first husband had dropped dead over his lathe in the factory where he worked; that her second husband drank too much, and that because her first had been a good one, she'd assumed that her second would be the same, that he (the second) had a wicked tongue, and hadn't any time for her now she'd got arthritis.

'Men are all the same,' said Miss Evans, and was

obviously all set to tell me that she'd once been kissed behind the Odeon, when an orderly walked past the doorway, her feet slapping on the polished floor in her crêpe-soled shoes, and Miss Evans stopped speaking as abruptly as if she'd been a radio and switched herself off.

I lay on my side and stared through the window. It was still raining, and a gust of wind blew spattering drops against the pane. Myrtle's bloomers, a pair of pink and a pair of blue, festooned the chipped radiator, Miss Evans sighed and said 'Dear God', and a woman in the next room started to cough.

It was two o'clock in the afternoon, and already the day seemed to have lasted for a week, but somewhere outside my mental Pollyanna must have peeped from behind the dripping rhododendrons, because I suddenly saw the funny side of things.

I made up my mind that I would never tell Frank, or anyone for that matter, just how awfully depressing that hospital was. My letters to him would be gay and care-free, the kind of letters he'd loved to receive all during the war.

And I kept my promise to myself, because until he read this account, more than twenty years afterwards, he had no idea, and when he'd finished reading it through, he put down the typed pages and looked at me thoughtfully, but he didn't say anything.

I was convalescing at the time, after yet another spell in hospital, this time after having had a steel plate inserted in my knee, jacking up the frayed edges of the joint.

'I'll go and make a coffee,' I told him, and leaving my walking stick dangling from the end of the sofa, I went into the kitchen, staggering a bit like a drunken sailor, but getting there on my own two good feet.

'We've been lucky, haven't we, love?' he said, and I knew exactly what he meant.

In spite of everything, that wheelchair was still a long

way away on the horizon.

'You bet,' I said.

And in spite of my initial reaction to the depressing atmosphere of the specialist hospital, Sheila had been right when she'd said they knew what they were doing. Ruthless the staff might be, and downright callous, it seemed to me at times, but what they were doing was to discipline us, and show us the kind of life, a rather restricted life, we ought to lead when we were sent out to face the world again.

It would take courage, the doctor told me at one of my weekly interviews with him, but not nearly the courage it would take to face life as a cripple. In common with most hospitals, they were short-staffed, and I seemed to spend my entire time, when I wasn't having treatments, wheeling old ladies to the lavatory, since their bladders refused to conform to the set times allotted to them by the orderlies.

Their pathetic gratitude knew no bounds, and I heard so many heart-rending stories of loneliness and rejection that I came to the conclusion that love as a commodity must be in very short supply.

It was almost like being in Retreat, and as the days slipped into weeks, I found that I was worrying less and less about my family outside. I just went for my treatments at the specified times, lay on my bed and rested when told to, ate when summoned by the gong, and after the first night, when I'd listened to Miss Evans saying 'Dear God' at half hourly intervals, slept for nine hours each night.

The doctor said that the ideal solution for arthritics would be for them to retire to a simple life, free from tension and bustle, but as that was not possible, a more rational solution would be to slow down our own style of living.

Big Annie, down in the treatment rooms, was a positive mine of information. In between wielding her hose-pipe, she told me to eat leafy vegetables every day, and that white sugar and bread would poison my whole system and lead to an early demise.

When I told her that my father-in-law put four spoonfuls in each cup of tea, and had never had a day's illness in his life, she completely ignored me, and went on to tell me that central heating was essential for anyone with arthritis, which was a BIG LAUGH, as Sheila would have said. I thought about our big cold house, with its unheated bedrooms, single coal fire in the living-room, and concrete floor in the kitchen, then obediently allowed myself to be half-lifted out of my shallow trough and stood for a few minutes underneath a cold shower to speed up my flagging circulation.

Sunbathing was very bad for inflamed joints, the kind young nurse in charge of the ultra-violet lamp told us, as we sat there in a circle, wearing brief shorts and dark spectacles, and I knew I could give up sunbathing without so much as a single qualm.

Possessing a fair skin, but still wanting to acquire a fashionable tan, I remembered the hours of holiday time I'd wasted, lying in the sun, watching with something akin to rage as Frank took on a flattering copper tone simply by sitting in the shade, and I merely freckled or burned. Now I had the perfect excuse for remaining a veritable English rose . . .

Big Annie told me they were going to try to 'sweat the arthritis out of me' . . . .

For those who can remember Marie Dressler in *Tugboat Annie*, she bore an uncanny resemblance to the long dead film star, and as she lowered me, none too gently, into a peat bath, I reckoned that working so long amid all that steam had given her a sadistic streak, along with a complexion as red and ruddy as a technicolor sunset.

The peat was black, and smelt disgusting. I had to lie in it for half an hour, breaking up with my hands the nauseating lumps, by way of exercise for my fingers.

After a necessary shower, Big Annie would wrap me in blankets and leave me lying on a couch in a cubicle, literally running with sweat.

'I may not go home cured,' I told Sheila, 'but at least I'll know I'm clean. To while away the two hours between supper and early bed-time, we started in training as table-tennis champions.

To say I am not sports-minded is perhaps the understatement of the year. I remember once walking to the library during the playing of extra-time in the World Cup final. The avenues were deserted, pails of water standing abandoned by cars in drives, entire families closeted behind closed curtains, watching television. I didn't meet a single soul, and in the library, the assistant stamped my books any old how, scuttling back to her transistor radio. I am, Frank tells me, totally incapable of keeping my eye on the ball!

We must have made an incongruous pair. Me hobbling about on my side of the table, making indecisive swipes with my little bat, both of us with our wrists encased in plaster, lunging at the ball, and Sheila swearing like a fish-wife when she missed.

'C'mon, honey,' she'd shout, when the score was nine games to two. 'You're not concentrating!'

They believed at that time that arthritis could be caused by germs which lodge in various organs of the body, and I was asked if I'd mind having my tonsils out.

I had the feeling it was going to be a process of elimination, and that they would progress from there to my gall-bladder, appendix, teeth, and anything else expendable, so I said I would give the matter my serious consideration. In the meantime, they started me on a course of penicillin injections, given by a nurse who could have passed for Big Annie's mother.

I had to report to the medical room three times a week, stand in a corner with my bottom bared to the elements, whilst she charged at me with a hypodermic needle. It didn't cure my arthritis, but it gave me an inborn mistrust of any nurse who smiles at me and says, 'Just a little prick now, dear.'

Frank came over to see me one weekend, bringing with him a snap of the girls looking long-legged and beautiful in his mother's garden, wearing their shorts and tee-shirts and wistful smiles.

He took Sheila and me out to tea in a nearby pub, and she flirted with him, and told him, much to his gratification, that he was the first real man she'd seen in months.

She looked magnificent in a scarlet linen suit, mini-skirted, long before they were the fashion, and I watched with amusement as Frank glowed as she fluttered her eyelashes at him. She'd told me of her many conquests, and in spite of the fact that she walked with a shuffle, and the deformity of her hands, she had a magnetic, almost animal appeal for men.

At least two of the porters were under her vivacious spell, and even the seriously dedicated doctor would stop and talk to her at every opportunity.

When she'd gone, leaving us with a suggestive wink, I plied Frank with questions about the girls, and he told me they were settling down happily again with Mrs Barlowe, and that everything was just fine.

I told him that I was just fine too, and when he caught his train, I walked slowly back to the hospital, feeling that he'd taken my heart with him, and wondering how I could endure another month away from them all.

Miss Evans told me that she'd seen us through the window, and what a nice young couple we made, and how glad she was that she'd never married, because she simply couldn't have borne to be a BURDEN to her husband.

Myrtle was having one of her 'off' days, and sat there on the edge of her bed, her fat legs wide apart, showing her pink bloomers.

'They've told me I can go home next week,' she said, 'but I know *he* don't want me back. He don't say. He isn't that bad, but I know he don't.'

I tried to comfort her.

'But you can't help having arthritis, Myrtle. And when you marry someone, you marry them for better or worse, and we could have far worse things wrong with us, you know.'

'Such as?' asked Myrtle.

'You must learn to smile through your tears,' said Miss Evans, 'the way I've taught myself to do. Pain is always sent to us for a purpose, you know.'

'That's stupid,' I couldn't help saying. 'Arthritis is a virus; we've just been unlucky, that's all, and look at Sheila. She has two children to bring up on her own, and no money, and she smiles all the time, and I don't mean through her tears, she just smiles.'

Miss Evans sniffed. 'I don't know how you can be so friendly with her. Common, that's what she is, and no better than she should be, if you ask me. Sex mad, I'd say.'

'And what's wrong with sex?' I asked them. I left them to their deflating conversation, and went in search of Sheila in the lounge.

The perpetual cigarette dangled from her mouth as she knitted furiously at the purple sweater, and I sat down beside her and stared at the glowing embers of the fire.

I imagined Frank in the train taking him back to the house in the Crescent, picking up the girls from a friend's house on the way, making their bedtime cocoa, putting them to bed, then studying alone in the living-room, his textbooks spread out on the dining-room table.

'Miss Evans says we must smile through our tears,' I said at last.

Sheila said that word again, and started on a purl row . . . .

At the end of the seventh week of daily treatment and long periods of rest, the doctor told me that my blood tests showed that the disease was much 'quieter' than when I was admitted. He said he would like me to stay for another three weeks, and reluctantly I agreed, only to receive, the very next morning, a letter from a friend who mentioned quite casually that Katy was ill.

'I met Frank on his way to the chemists to buy his third bottle of calamine lotion,' she wrote. 'He says poor wee Katy keeps him awake all night, and is scratching herself raw.'

I sat on the edge of my bed, reading and re-reading the letter. Chicken-pox never crossed my mind, so sure was I that Katy had some awful, mind-induced skin disease; small-pox at the very least, then I reassured myself with the thought that she was at home scratching her little body raw, instead of in some isolation hospital.

'Bad news, dear?' asked Miss Evans hopefully.

'I'm going home tomorrow,' I told her, and went downstairs to the surgery to request an appointment with the doctor.

Sheila had gone home the week before, armed with a list of instructions I knew she would never keep.

'Think of me sometimes, honey,' she'd said, 'and don't do anything I wouldn't do – that gives you plenty of scope.'

She walked to the station, carrying her heavy case, still bare-legged, her blond hair, with its wide black parting, skewered to the top of her head. I would have gone with her, but I was due for a session with Big Annie, and Sheila turned to wave at me, twiddling her red-tipped fingers and smiling, still smiling.

I missed her very much. Myrtle had gone home also, back to the husband who no longer wanted her, and her bed had been taken by a patient with arthritis in her spine.

Poker-spine, she told us, a condition where the verte-brae grow together, making the back as rigid as a steel pole. She informed us that her spine was stiffening day by day; that she could actually *feel* it stiffening by the hour, and her depression lifted Miss Evans's spirits wonderfully.

They got on famously together, outdoing each other in reporting imaginative symptoms to Sister on her round. They were so miserable, so enamoured with their suffering, I felt genuinely guilty about my own improvement in health.

I had put on half a stone in weight, my hair shone, and the dull yellow glaze had gone from my eyes. True, my left knee was still badly swollen, my ankles ached, and my wrists sent stabbing pains up my arms if I attempted to do anything more strenuous than turn the pages of a book, but I was more than ready to take on the running of my home again.

I told the doctor this, and although I knew he couldn't stop me from discharging myself, I expected a lecture about ungrateful patients who terminated their treatments before time.

Instead, he listened patiently, whilst I painted a highly dramatic picture of Katy sobbing piteously for her mother during the long watches of the night.

He heard me out, then, leaning forward, clasping his hands together on his blotting pad, he told me that I could go home the coming Saturday, only two days away.

I thanked him for all that had been done for me, and as so many doctors have done since then, he waved my thanks aside.

'Rest, and more rest,' he reminded me, and I promised on my honour that I'd sleep ten hours each night, and spend my afternoons in bed with a good book.

In order to be allowed to go home I'd have promised him I'd lie down for twenty-three hours out of the twenty-four, spending the hour I was up doing exercises, and by the twinkle in his eyes, I realized he knew this.

'Good luck,' he said, and actually got up from his desk and came round and shook my hand.

He was watching my face carefully, waiting, I felt sure, for me to wince as he gripped my fingers in his firm clasp, but I smiled straight into his rather beautiful brown eyes through the unexpected prick of tears behind my own.

Miss Evans would have been proud of me . . . .

# 8

The next important thing was to let Frank know that I would be coming home so, in between a session underneath an infra-red lamp positioned so that it shone on the back of my neck, and a date with Big Annie down in the treatment rooms, I managed to fit in a telephone call to my neighbour.

I could see her standing there in the hall of her pin-neat home, so clean and cherished that there was a little potted plant on a lace doily atop her washing machine, and a knitted crinoline lady covering the spare toilet roll in the lavatory.

'Frank must borrow our car,' she said at once, 'and come and fetch you himself. You can't come alone by train, lugging a case, and undoing all the good that's been done to you. No, I absolutely insist, love, you must have our car.'

Kindness always takes me unawares, destroying all my defences, and I went down to Big Annie so overcome that I had to blurt out my news straightaway.

I didn't tell her that Katy was ill, and that I'd discharged myself; I didn't dare, not when she was standing over me as I lay in the shallow bath, wielding the hose-pipe with its fierce jet of water straight at my anatomy.

I felt she might have directed it into my eye for being so stupid!

As it was, she said it was sudden news, wasn't it? And how come she hadn't noticed that my name hadn't been struck from her list?

'You wouldn't go and do a foolish thing like discharging yourself now, would you?' she asked, her small piggy eyes shining through the all-enveloping steam.

'Do you think I'd do a thing like that?' I murmured, closing my eyes. Then I spent the half hour when I should have been relaxing, listening for the slap of her boat-sized crêpe shoes approaching my cubicle.

She couldn't kill me, I kept telling myself, not convincing myself one little bit!

Miss Evans told me I wasn't being fair to my husband, and that she just hoped he'd understand, that was all.

So did I, but for the time being, all that mattered was that I was going home. That in less than two days' time, *I* would be the one who dabbed Katy's spots with calamine lotion, and comforted her when she itched.

That Saturday morning, my breakfast of sausage, bacon and tomatoes stuck in my throat, and I pushed my plate away. At 8.30 I positioned myself by the window of my room, staring down at the circular drive, my case packed and ready, willing the car to appear.

Miss Evans had been wheeled away for X-rays, and the lady with the poker-spine was fast asleep, snoring gently, her lower lip shuddering with each rise and fall of breath, her hands crossed over the lace front of her nightie. I wished her well; I wished everyone in that big impersonal barn of a hospital well, but I knew that after a week back home, I would be giving them no more than a reluctant, passing thought.

I left a box of chocolates with a little note on Miss Evans's bed, then I went and sat too near the radiator, feeling the perspiration beading my upper lip. But nothing could have made me move from my vantage point, and I glanced at my watch, at what I was sure were half hourly intervals, only to be astonished each time to find that only ten minutes had passed by.

By ten o'clock, I was telling myself that Frank had got the message wrong; that he had thought I had said Sunday, and by 10.30, I was sure he had been involved in an accident, and actually saw him hunched over the steering wheel, our kindly neighbour's car a complete write-off.

The lady with the poker-spine was propped up in bed to drink her coffee, but I refused to go downstairs for mine. It was as though I was growing from that radiator, and when I saw the blue car turn into the drive, I picked up my case, and ran as fast as my gammy knee would let me, down the wide staircase.

I'd said my goodbyes, expressed my thanks, and as I raced past the little porter behind his desk, he gave me the thumbs-up sign, and I stepped out into the blinding sunshine of a glorious summer's day.

And there was Frank, and there, in the back of the car, were the girls. Wide-eyed with excitement, Katy with her little heart-shaped face dotted with scabs, her beloved suck-a-blanket cradled in her arms.

They had obviously been given strict instructions to stay where they were, so I got into the car, kneeling up on the front seat, and gathered them close to me. Marilyn said dramatically:

'I promised Daddy I wouldn't cry, and I'm not going to.'

Katy just stared at me, picking at a sore place on the bridge of her nose.

'She has chicken-pox,' Frank told me, unnecessarily, 'but she's much better, and the doctor said it wouldn't do her any harm to have a bit of fresh air, as long as she didn't come into contact with anyone.'

'Can you skip now, Mummy?' Marilyn asked me, and I said we'd see the moment we got home. Katy insisted on coming in the front with me, sitting on my knee, and I held her tight, feeling my very heart dissolving with love and happiness. I stared at her spotty little face, and thought how worried, and yes, *surprised* she looked, how surprised they both looked, until I realized that Frank had plaited their brown hair so tightly that their eyebrows had been pulled up into expressions of perpetual astonishment.

'I haven't had time to do the weekend shopping,' Frank told me, and I said it didn't matter. I was in charge again, and nothing mattered, and as we drove along we saw a goat tethered to a grassy bank, so we stopped the car, and wound down the windows to watch it.

'I'm on Book Five now,' Marilyn told me, and Katy said she'd been all itchy, but now she wasn't, and I told Frank about the letter from my friend, and confessed I'd asked to be sent home.

For a moment he looked angry. 'That wasn't very wise, was it?' he said, and I told him that I'd never considered myself to be particularly wise, and I'd come to the conclusion that I was one of those nauseating mothers who would crawl through fire and flood-water to be with their nearest and dearest.

'How could you crawl when you can't even kneel down?' asked Frank, and I knew he'd forgiven me, and wouldn't refer to it again.

The first thing Marilyn did when we arrived back home, even before I'd switched on the kettle for the cup of really hot tea I'd been dreaming about, was to fetch her skipping ropes from the toy drawer in the kitchen, and pull me by the hand out on to the lawn.

Katy, still dragging her filthy blanket, followed, and as I hesitated, I saw Frank, through the window, giving me the thumbs-up sign from the sink where he was washing up their breakfast things.

A red wooden handle in each hand, I glanced with apprehension at the long length of rope. To walk? Yes, that was possible, even with a limp. To run? Yes, even that, in my own fashion. But to skip?

Then I saw Marilyn's round freckled face, and knew that to her a Mummy who could skip was a Mummy restored fully to health once again. Proof positive of my return to mobility.

So slowly at first, then with increasing confidence, sending up a silent prayer of thanks to all the doctors and nurses back at the hospital, not forgetting Big Annie, I turned the ropes, and there on the daisy spattered lawn, I began to skip . . . .

The improvement in my condition lasted for almost a year after the long summer I'd spent resting and having specialized treatment. I knew now how to cope with arthritis, and without considering myself in the least an invalid, I recognized my limitations, and rested more.

I even bought a pair of shoes with *heels*, flashy ones, court style, with a bow on their fronts. I couldn't walk any distance outside in them, but it was good just to own them, and wear them when I was all dressed up, and friends came to call.

I loved just sitting there, feeling feminine once again, with my ankles neatly crossed to show them off, hoping my friends had noticed them. The fact that I had to kick them off when I went through into the kitchen to make coffee passed without comment, and although I never actually skipped again, I prided myself on being able to walk without too much of a list to starboard.

Then one day Frank came home and told me that he'd got a chance of a job in Birmingham, a promotion, and was going for an interview the following week.

'How would you feel about leaving Lancashire?'

'I wouldn't mind in the least,' I said, 'it will be a fresh start.'

'Do we *need* a fresh start?' asked Frank, ever practical, and completely impervious to my dramatic turn of speech.

He got the job, as I'd told him he would. He said that he'd have to live in digs whilst he looked around for a house, and we worked out that the very small deposit we could afford qualified us for a down payment on a tent, or at best a rickety caravan.

'We'll find something,' I assured him, and waved him off one bitterly cold morning, around the time when dawn was just beginning to crack. His going had wakened the girls, and when I went back to bed, they crept in with

90

me, and we huddled together in our icy cold bedroom, and I told them tales about how they'd love living in Birmingham, and would make lots of new friends, and what a big place it was.

As I'd never been there myself, my descriptions were a bit vague, but I said there was bound to be a zoo, complete with red-bottomed monkeys, like the ones in London.

'I won't like it if Pat can't come. She's my very best friend, and I'll cry if I have to leave her,' said Marilyn, staring sadly over the sheet into a depressing vista of the unknown.

'I'm not going,' Katy said simply, and started to cough, a funny little cough, which ended on a frightening whoop.

I asked her to cough again, and she obliged, this time seeming to hold her breath until her face turned purple.

'Has anyone at school got whooping cough?' I asked, and Marilyn assured me that simply everyone had whooping cough; that her classroom was filled with boys and girls whooping their hearts out over their desks, and that the girl sitting next to her had been sick on Book Seven only the previous Friday.

'But *I'm* on Book Nine,' she went on. 'It doesn't matter being the worst at sums if you're the best at reading, does it? I hope I have whooping cough, because then I won't be able to go to Birmingham and leave Pat. She's only on Book Eight.'

Her wish was granted, and the following weekend, Frank came home to a house reeking of wintergreen, and two daughters coughing and being sick with alternating regularity.

The housing situation was hopeless, he told me. There was just nothing we could afford, and I didn't add to his worry by telling him that my arthritic symptoms had come back with a vengeance, in all the places previously affected, and in addition, swelling up my big-toe joints like massive bunions, and making the wearing of shoes agony.

My beautiful court shoes with their pretty bows on front had long since been relegated to the back of the wardrobe, and I was back to wearing sandals in summer, and boots a size too big in winter.

My lovely coalman had let me have two extra bags of coal, and I had been struggling to carry buckets upstairs to light a fire in the bedroom grate which belched black smoke and made the girls cough even more. Frank went into town, and came back with a small electric radiator. He would go off to Birmingham at six o'clock on the Monday morning, leaving Katy and Marilyn warm but still coughing.

Four months later, when their whoops were a thing of the past, he was still doing the rounds of the estate agents in Birmingham's suburbs, trying to find a house we could afford.

Then one evening, my kindly neighbour came round to tell me that he was on the telephone, and I went with her, knowing that only something of great importance would have induced him to trade on her good nature in this way.

'I've found a house,' he said, 'very small, but with a garden. Can you come down tomorrow? We have to decide straight away.'

'Yes,' I said promptly, and fixed up for Marilyn to stay with her beloved Pat, and for Katy to go to friends round the corner.

I hadn't travelled by train alone for a long time, mainly because trains have handles on their doors that I can't manipulate. I always imagined myself being carried on to Carlisle or even further when all I wanted was the next station but one.

But this time I had no choice, and as I sat there, in a not over-crowded compartment, praying that someone would be getting out at Birmingham, I decided that unless the house had no roof and backed on to the gas-works, I would say I liked it.

Frank was waiting for me, and we caught a bus out to

the Coventry side of Birmingham, a journey which took roughly twenty minutes. We got off the bus, crossed the road, and started to walk up a long, winding road. Frank said it wasn't far.

'How far?' I asked, after we'd been walking for about a quarter of an hour, my knee aching in angry protest.

I could sense that he was rather worried.

'It didn't *seem* to be this far, and I don't remember that farm, nor those cows. I had the impression it was houses all the way.'

We trudged on for another five minutes without speaking.

The houses, identical to the last grain of grey pebble dash, started again, square, small, devoid of the least sign of character, with front gardens no bigger than a hop and a jump. For those who *could* hop and jump, I amended silently.

'Did you by any chance come out by car?' I asked, and Frank admitted that a friend had given him a lift, then rounding a bend he stopped suddenly, pointing a triumphant finger.

'That's it, love! At the top of this next short incline, on the right.'

I stared with disbelief into the far distance. It was like looking at a drawing, the kind I'd been so bad at at school, where two lines appear to grow together in the distance, the far, far distance. I said not a word, because I was thinking of all the weeks he'd searched for a place not far removed from our previous style of living, and when at last we rang the door bell of a house with a turquoise door and were invited inside by a young woman who looked as fresh as H.E. Bates' Watercress Girl, I was glad I'd kept quiet.

The house, although minute, was as warm and cosy as a haybox, and the hall was just about big enough for two people to stand side by side. There was a tiny lounge, a smaller dining-room, and a narrow kitchen, beautifully work-studied by the simple expedient of being so narrow that by standing at the sink and stretching out a hand, everything was there, within easy reach.

There were two bedrooms, and a bathroom with a lavatory as part of the bright turquoise suite, with a candlewick cover on the seat, and bath-mat, towels, and face-cloths, all in the same shade. I concluded it must have been the owner's favourite colour!

'How far away are we from shops, and a school?' I asked her, sinking gratefully into the chair she offered when our tour of inspection was over, and she told me they were both 'quite a walk away', but that groceries could be delivered.

Frank reminded me that I had a bike, and the girls two good legs apiece, and seeing his worried face, I said it was lovely, and that I was sure we'd manage.

'My wife has arthritis,' he explained, and the Water-cress Girl asked me had I ever tried apple cider vinegar . . . .

We stayed the night in Frank's digs, sleeping together in a bed so narrow that we had to turn over in unison, and in the morning, without the comfort of my customary hot bath, I was so stiff I could only just hobble down-stairs, and his landlady asked me had I ever tried the peanut cure . . . .

Back home I told the girls about the house, and that they would be sharing a room, and because at that time they were going through a phase of actually liking each other, they greeted my news with rapturous delight.

The exchanging of contracts and all the preliminaries of buying a house went through without a hitch. We said goodbye to all our friends and relatives, watched all our furniture being loaded into a van, and caught the train to Birmingham.

I had been busy cutting down curtains to size, and we weren't sure how our furniture would fit in, but of one thing we were certain. Everything would be too big.

I was determined not to worry. Being an arthritic makes you get things into perspective, and besides, worry was bad for me. The doctor had told me so.

But my hard-won passivity was put to the test when the furniture van failed to turn up.

Our worldly goods were in that van, all we possessed in the world, and when after four days it hadn't materialized, I felt that even the doctor would have allowed me one small niggle of doubt that we would ever see it again . . . .

'Thanks be to goodness Katy brought her suck-a-blanket with her on the train,' said Marilyn, as we bedded them down for the third night running on the wide sofa in the living-room of Frank's digs.

'Or else I would be really worried,' said Katy . . . .

# 9

Whenever I read in a newspaper that some luckless family has been left with 'only the clothes they stand up in', I *identify*.

'Lost in transit' was the only explanation we were ever given, and when the van did turn up on the fourth day, I had to go out into the road and touch it, to make sure it was really there.

It wasn't the loss of all our furniture and carpets which worried me, but trivial, personal things, like the holiday snaps of the girls when they were babies, my vast collection of books, and Frank's pipe-rack, which he'd made when he was a boy.

We'd had to throw ourselves on the mercy of his landlady, and I tried to make it sound like an adventure, but Marilyn said she didn't like adventures, and never had, and Katy said if she didn't get her new pencil-box back, she would die . . . .

I asked Frank if we were insured, and he said of course we were, and I cheered up a little, and imagined us going into a big store in Birmingham, and ordering a replacement of everything, from Katy's pencil-box to a three-piece suite.

'My mind's boggling,' I said, and Frank said his was wobbling a bit too.

We went to the pictures one afternoon, just to take our minds off it, and Marilyn cried all through a wide-screen version of *The Robe*, and Katy went to sleep. Afterwards we walked up the long road to our new and empty house, and stood around on the bare floorboards wondering what to do next.

When the van did arrive at last, we were dirty, dis-illusioned, but grateful beyond words, and soon found out that we'd been right in our assumption that every-thing would be too big.

Cramming two single beds in the girls' room left just about enough space for an undersized skeleton to walk between them, and I swore I wouldn't mind having to climb over my washing-machine to get to the sink. But by cutting carpets in half, and deciding we'd have to keep the dining-room table permanently folded, we finally considered ourselves moved in.

The girls started attending a school of more than a thousand pupils, walking a mile to get there, a complete contrast to their little village school in Lancashire. Frank left home half an hour earlier each morning to walk to the station, and I clocked up more miles on my bicycle riding to the shops than if I'd been training for the Tour de France.

I found a doctor's surgery. He took one look at me and passed me on to the nearest hospital only five miles away, and told me to register there as an out-patient.

Quite conditioned by now to going two miles for a postage stamp, I set off for my first appointment, riding to a bus stop, leaving my bicycle leaning up against the railings of a big house, then taking the bus the rest of the way.

For the two years we were to live in Birmingham, that my bicycle was still there each time where I'd left it, unpadlocked, seemed to prove two things. One that the people of the Midlands are honest to a man, or that my precious bike was so rusty and dilapidated, it just wasn't worth the pinching!

At the hospital, I went once again through the routine of blood-tests, X-rays, and examinations; was told to attend monthly, step up the aspirins, rest more, eat more, and not to worry.

A refined-looking lady in the waiting-room told me

that part of the country was the worst spot for arthritis and chests. I told her we'd just moved down from Lancashire again, and she said she'd known that as soon as I'd opened my mouth.

I resolved never to say words like bus and butter again . . . .

Because we knew no one, and had no baby-sitter, we hardly went out at all. As our finances improved, we bought our first television set, and spent the evenings glued to it, watching the test card with rapt attention, and only exchanging odd bits of conversation during the interludes.

Frank had a colleague at work whose family was living in Liverpool. He would come round on Wednesdays, seat himself silently on the sofa as we goggled in the warm gloom, and go to catch his last bus before we switched off and went to bed.

'If I saw you in the light, I doubt if I'd recognize you,' I told him once, and was instantly shushed into silence, as the next item was introduced.

The little house was so cosy, I don't remember being cold once during the time we lived there. I was told at the hospital that gentle heat increased the circulation, bringing healing blood to the inflamed joints, and so we bought an infra-red lamp, and I spent many happy hours in its glow.

I've learnt since that infra-red lamps do no more than soothe, and can indeed do harm if used too often; that *ice* is often better. That may be true, but on one of my visits to the hospital I was told I had to wear a collar (a high plaster-cast) to relieve the severe pain I was getting up the back of my head, but I persevered with the lamp, and managed without the collar.

I shone it on my hands as I sewed dresses for the girls, I shone it on my feet as I read a book, and looking back, I seem to have spent those two years basking in its lovely warmth.

Then Frank came home one day, and told me he was

going down to London for an interview, and I was surprised to find just how much I'd miss our little doll's house. Its disadvantages had been many, but we'd been very happy there.

True, the inconvenience of having the lavatory in the bathroom meant that one of the girls always wanted to 'go', just as Frank started to shave, but we were all excited, especially Katy, who was sure that living near London meant she would see the Queen every day.

This time there wouldn't be the problem of him finding rooms, as his parents lived in Hatch End, a spreading suburb which had not all that long ago been a country village. And this time, having a house to sell, we wouldn't have the traumatic experience of trying to scrape up a deposit.

He was there only a matter of weeks before he found a house in a tree-lined avenue, bordering on the green belt, with a school round the corner, and a mere five minutes' walk away from a splendid boulevard of shops.

This time our furniture actually turned up on time. Now we were faced with the problem of not having enough to go round, finding that curtains didn't fit, and that carpets left wide borders of unpolished floorboards.

I made the mistake of trying to kneel down to stain them dark oak, and my knees rebelled so badly that one of them swelled to the size of a prize cabbage at a horticultural show, and I made the now all too familiar journey to a doctor's surgery.

He was a Scot, with eyes of a vivid blue, as handsome as Doctor Finlay, but without his aggressive manner. I wasn't surprised when he gave me a letter to take to the 'local' hospital, a mere four miles away as the crow flies, but necessitating catching two buses and a train.

Because I could barely walk, it was arranged that I had transport, so three times a week an ambulance would call for me, and I would climb in amongst the local arthritics, victims of strokes and worse, and be taken on a circular tour of the whole area, before arriving at the hospital where they shone a lamp on me exactly like the one I had at home, only bigger.

The whole morning would be taken up with ten minutes heat treatment, and I told the young physiotherapist that I could do the same at home, plus practising the exercises, which I'd been doing for years anyway.

'These lamps should only be used under supervision,' I was told firmly. So, because I am not the militant type and would never sit on my bottom in Trafalgar Square, however worthy the cause, I submitted, and went weekly for my sessions, wasting, I was convinced, three whole mornings, but too passive-minded to make a stand.

The arthritis, although I would never have admitted it, grew steadily worse over the next few years. I remember going into town one Christmas to buy presents, walking round a big store, catching sight of myself in a mirror, and being amazed to see a middle-aged thirty-five-year-old woman staring back at me, hair straggling, face more transparent than pale, wearing boots a size too big, and with an expression of such exhaustion that I recoiled.

I'd stuck to my maxim of not letting my family suffer with me, and the girls grew up just as selfish, just as inconsiderate, just as lovable as any other adolescents. They had lost any trace of their Lancashire accents, and talked 'posh', like southerners born and bred.

'I wish you wouldn't say bath, Mummy,' Katy, now Kate, told me one day. 'It's barth.'

'And it's grars, not grass.' Marilyn admonished; I told them I was too old to change, and they'd just have to put up with me.

I joined the Young Wives belonging to the church, and when I was too long in the tooth, the Mother's Union. I rode down to the hall on my bicycle, and went to coffee mornings, knowing all the time that there was something somewhere, surely, that I could do with my time which would give me greater satisfaction.

'I'm the creative type,' I told Frank, 'and if I knew I

could get there in the mornings, I'd find myself a job.'

'I'm a cabbage,' I told him, as countless wives of growing families have told their husbands, and he listened, puffing at his pipe, and asked me why I didn't have the nice girl down the road in for tea, as she looked just my type.

'But that's just it. She *isn't* my type at all,' I exploded. 'She only wants to talk about which washing powder she uses, and repeat the cute sayings of her children, and our two never say anything cute. Never.'

'You couldn't possibly do a job as well as run the house,' Frank told me quietly, and I knew that he was right.

So I made my now monthly visits to the hospital, braving the long journey by buses and train rather than ride in the tumbril, as I called the ambulance; stayed at home, struggled through the housework in my own fashion, knowing that if only I could find the key, there was *something* I could do.

One evening, as we watched television, me reading a magazine by the light of a table lamp at the same time, I finished a story and turned to Frank.

'I bet I could write a story if I tried,' I said, and Frank slewed his eyes away from the flickering screen long enough to grin at me.

'You need more experience of life than you've had, love, to write,' he told me, and I bit my lip, but nodded in agreement.

'I suppose you're right,' I admitted slowly, and sighing, picked up another magazine.

By this time we owned a car, and this of course meant mobility for me, but only when Frank was at the wheel.

'I'll learn to drive,' I said.

My aunt was staying with us at the time, for her annual summer visit, and in her forthright Lancashire way, told me that I'd never manage it, not with my hands.

'But people drive cars who have only one arm. And no

legs!' I said, for good measure.

Then Frank, a dedicated engineer, with as much respect for what goes on underneath the bonnet of a car as a surgeon has for what lies inside a human body, explained to me that I would never manage the gears; that because of my right arm I could never give hand signals, and that my feet weren't pliant enough to manipulate the pedals. I was forced to see their point of view.

I was increasingly aware of the fact that I was an arthritic, a *disabled person*, and during the week, my only outlet from the house was when I rode my bicycle to the shops, and even doing that was becoming more and more difficult, as I found the brakes almost impossible to manage.

During the long, sunny afternoons, I went out into the garden, trying to do a little gentle weeding. Knowing, but only just, the difference between a blade of grass and a clump of lilies of the valley, this was in itself a chancy business, but at least it was a hobby, and got me out into the fresh air.

It wasn't long before I had to give this up, however. Bending made my back ache, and pulling up weeds started up the pain in my hands again. I went back to my sewing-machine, making dresses for Marilyn, now rapidly approaching her teens, only to be told, with actual tears in her eyes, that I had no idea of *style*, and that she'd rather die than go out with her friends in the creations I ran up for her.

There were no such problems with Kate, now in her first year at a grammar school. She had already developed a style of her own. A style which consisted of being clad from throat to ankles in deep black; black sweaters, black slacks, with eyeliner to tone, and I turned my frustrated creative urges to doing crossword puzzles.

Words fascinated me, and I wasted hours poring over crossword puzzles with fiendish clues, even taking them with me to the hospital to while away the hours waiting for treatment. One day I was sent to see a doctor I had never seen before, and when I told him I was seething with a mass of frustrations, even if it didn't show, and that the trek to the hospital was making me worse instead of better, he actually *listened* to me.

He was a big man, a huge kindly man, with hands like hams, which I felt sure must have had the healing touch. He agreed with me about the exercises and the lamp, and told me he was going to start me on a course of cortisone.

Cortisone was first derived from ox-bile, but it is now possible to synthesize the substance. It is produced by the adrenal gland, and in its early stages was hailed as a wonder drug. It will not heal a damaged joint, and the lost cartilage or bone surface will not return. The side-effects can include indigestion, flushing, and most patients, even those taking small doses, develop a chubbiness of the face, called Moon-face.

If a patient taking the drug has an accident, or has to undergo surgery, or develops pneumonia, it is important not to let the treatment lapse. In cases like this the dosage is increased temporarily, or alternatively the patient is given a few injections of hydrocortisone to help them over the period of 'stress'.

Another complication is that patients on cortisone must not stop the tablets suddenly, in case they develop withdrawal symptoms, so stopping them has to be done carefully and gradually under medical supervision.

But in cases which do not respond to ordinary treatment, with cortisone there is sometimes a remarkable improvement, and the disease is put into a state of artificial suppression.

All this was explained to me, in terms I could understand. I was told that my left knee, my right shoulder, and both my hands were damaged beyond the stage where cortisone could help, but my new doctor gave me HOPE, and I came home with my little bottle of tablets, feeling that now at last something beyond my own will-power was working for me.

I refused to consider that I might develop a fever, a bad stomach, spots, dizziness, irritated kidneys, plus a swollen and distorted face. What did any of these matter, if I could walk? So I swallowed them dutifully, and within *weeks*, or even days, I began to feel better.

Looking at snaps taken during the years I was on cortisone, I realize now that my face, always fairly round, did resemble the full moon, both in colour and shape, but no one was unkind enough to tell me, and I never did grow a moustache or hairs on my bosoms, other eventualities which had been suggested to me.

Before long I was actually able to leave my ancient bicycle at home and walk to the shops. I bought a shopping trolley, and joined the other matrons of Hatch End, dragging it behind me as I walked down the tree-lined avenues with as much pride as if I'd been taking out a new baby for the first time.

My new doctor injected rebellious joints with hydro-cortisone, drew off the fluid when my knee became too swollen for comfort, and one day suggested manipulation for an ankle.

The effect of manipulation is to restore use to joints, muscles, and tendons. By skilful pressure, the changed parts are set back into place, force never being used. The patient is given a general anaesthetic, as if for an operation, and for the next few days the joint is painful, but by removing the stress it can postpone the arthritic process, and get the patient back on her feet, even if only temporarily.

The girls, by now, were self-reliant, and able to take charge in an emergency. Kate cooked delicious meals, throwing in handfuls of herbs and spices. She was going through a domestic phase, and washing up a few cups and saucers entailed wiping down the kitchen walls, polishing the cooker until it shone, and using half a packet of soap powder to wash out the tea towel.

Marilyn, on the other hand, was a dreamy, willowy adolescent, with a liking for reading poetry aloud.

'You do understand, Mummy,' she said to me one day, 'that the mere sight of a wet dishcloth turns my stomach?'

Sitting there, with my newly manipulated ankle stretched out on a stool, I said that of course I understood, and obediently listened as her dark brown voice intoned a poem of Keats . . . .

'When I have fears that I may cease to be . . .' she read, as her younger sister's tousled head appeared round the sitting-room door.

'How long is it since you washed the kitchen curtains, Mummy?'

'About three months,' I whispered, closing my eyes as the beautiful words washed over me.

'No wonder they're absolutely filthy,' said Kate, and withdrew, the light of battle in her eye.

# 10

Although arthritis is not *caused* by the emotions, the mental state of a patient does have a big part to play in its progression, and when my kindly rheumatologist at the hospital told me on one of my now three-monthly visits (the cortisone making the longer time lapse possible) that a psychiatrist from Australia was working at the hospital, compiling a dossier on the cause and effects of arthritis, I was positively affronted when he suggested that I had an interview with him.

The idea that some quirk in my mentality could have been the cause of all those years of pain niggled, and when I mentioned this to the nurse in charge, she laughed out loud.

'But the doctor wants you to see him because of your unusually cheerful attitude to your complaint. He thinks that what you might have to say could help other people who are afflicted. He wants to know why you are able mentally to shrug off your disability, and what makes you tick.'

That was better. . . .

I imagined myself lying flat on a horsehair sofa, as in a television serial running at that time, whilst he sat by my head, pencil poised over a pad, taking down my every utterance. The very idea brought out the worst side of the exhibitionist in me, and I went quite gaily for my appointment.

I was a bit put off by the fact that there was no sofa, only a hard chair for me to sit on, across a desk from a young outdoor type of doctor, with a tape recorder switched on at the ready.

Eagerly I launched into a lurid description of my early days. My mother dying having me, my father walking away and deserting me, the privations of being a child who had never known either parent. I told him how I used to go and visit my paternal grandmother and stand on her doorstep counting to a hundred, willing my father to turn the corner of her road.

'You must realize that your father is married and has children of his own,' she told me one Sunday morning, as I stood there in the doorway, praying for the sight of the tall figure in a brown suit striding towards me.

'But *I* was his first baby,' I'd said, and giving full rein to my thwarted creative urges, I gave this little anecdote all I'd got.

To my surprise, the ruddy-cheeked doctor wasn't even mildly interested, actually stopping me in mid-flow with a raised brown hand.

'Just answer my questions, please,' he said.

Deciding he didn't know his job, and had no soul to boot, I waited meekly to hear again the question he'd already asked me, before I got launched into my own little private Peyton Place.

'What do you think has helped you most in your fight against arthritis?'

The side of me that loves to make outrageous remarks wanted to say: 'My own indomitable spirit, of course,' but I didn't think his sense of humour would be of the Lancashire variety, so I told what I felt to be the truth.

'My husband,' I said, trying to make my tones dulcet in deference to the tape recorder.

Immediately, the tanned young man brightened up.

'You mean he has helped around the house, and seen to it that you rested?'

'He has helped me by *not* helping me,' I said.

'How do you mean?' said my interrogator, obviously wondering what he'd done to deserve me.

I leaned forward confidently, enjoying every minute.

I'd come to enjoy myself, and by golly I was going to.

'He has never allowed me to feel that I am anything but a normal woman. He knows that if he stretches out a hand to help me, I am more than likely to knock it away. He boosts my morale by telling me I look good when I am tired, and he praises me when I complete a task that other normal women would take for granted.'

I was well into my stride by now.

'He doesn't rush forward to help me up out of chairs, because he knows I would hate it. And he swears that my hands aren't noticeable, so that just occasionally, if someone does mention them, and wonder aloud how I cope, I get a shock because quite honestly I never think about their shape.'

'That's very interesting,' said my interviewer, and after the tape was switched off, told me that my attitude was refreshing and unique, and when I got up to go, he shook hands with me so heartily that my arm-pits tingled, but after what he'd said I couldn't let myself down, so I smiled at him through set teeth, and said goodbye.

'I'm not a nut-case,' I told Frank that evening. 'I'm not even neurotic.'

'I could have told you that for nothing,' said Frank, and I smiled, knowing that to him nerves are just things that have to be pulled together, and never never indulged in.

My doctor was going on a lecture tour of America, and asked me to write a paper, putting down how I faced up to my disabilities. When I'd finished it read like a cross between Little Orphan Annie and a Patience Strong sampler. I imagined it being read over all networks right across the States, and my own stock went up no end.

The cortisone was giving me back my belief in myself, a confidence I'd been in danger of losing, and we started going out more with friends. I bought a long dress, my first, my chance having been lost because of the war, and I actually danced!

Not the Gay Gordons to be sure, and with summer sandals on my feet instead of the silver-strapped sandals my soul yearned for, but dancing all the same.

I'll never forget the first time I danced in the warm gloom of a London night club. Leaning on my partner, and shuffling round the tiny floor, with the music sending shivers of pure delight up and down my spine. I remember closing my eyes and clutching my surprised, but nonetheless willing partner closer, and wondering just how any woman could take a moment like that for granted.

On one particular evening, Frank and I were to act as host and hostess, welcoming our guests as they came down the staircase of a famous Park Lane hotel, and shaking hands with them.

We'd discussed it all beforehand.

'But you can't shake hands with over a hundred people,' Frank said. 'Your hands couldn't take it.'

'I could stand behind you with a white glove on a stick,' said Kate. 'You know, poking it through underneath your arm.'

'You could wear your arm in a sling,' said Marilyn.

'Or have a placard on your chest, saying FRAGILE,' said Kate, on the verge of giggling hysteria.

'Or kiss all the men so passionately that their wives won't *want* to shake hands with you,' said Marilyn, not to be outdone.

'I will behave quite normally,' I said with dignity, and stood there by Frank's side, feeling my knees swelling there underneath my lovely new gown, and shaking hands with every single guest.

I regretted it the morning afterwards, but oh, how it was worth it, every precious painful minute. . . .

And along with my new-found, cortisone-instilled freedom came again the longing to 'prove' myself in some way. The urge to *express* myself.

But how?

The girls were growing up. They were both at grammar

schools, and Marilyn had joined the church youth club, being escorted home by a varied succession of boyfriends, each one, or so it seemed to us, more furtive and hairy than his predecessor.

I found myself bringing the facts of life casually into conversations, only to be asked why middle-aged people seemed to be so obsessed by sex?

One particular boyfriend, with the looks of Sasha Distel, and the morals, I convinced myself, of an alleycat, had a motor-bike. The first time I saw my lovely, sweet, and kind elder daughter climb on to the pillion, wind her arms round the unsavoury one's waist, to be borne away down the avenue at the speed of light, I went back into the house, swallowed another cortisone tablet, and started on a crossword, only to find that the simplest of clues was beyond me.

And in spite of the cortisone, my hands were becoming increasingly useless, bearing out the fact that even a miracle drug couldn't restore damaged joints.

I had managed to find a cleaning woman, a tiny bright-eyed lady who came on Fridays to do what I wasn't able to do – such as cleaning windows, mopping the kitchen floor, hard polishing, and making beds more thoroughly than by just flicking the blankets into place – the method I'd had to employ.

To say she was thorough would be the understatement of the year.

Although she weighs no more than seven stone, and has a damaged lung, she doesn't clean a room, she 'bottoms' it, flinging wardrobes around as if they are matchboxes. Her way of making a bed is to dismantle it, brushing the mattress and beating the pillows within an inch of their lives.

She is still with me, after all these years, and her coming meant that I had more time on my hands. More time to worry about Marilyn and her retinue of boyfriends, especially the current one, who seemed to spend all his time playing an imaginary guitar with one hand,

and caressing her with the other.

And more time to nourish the feeling that somewhere, sonehow, there was something I could do. . . .

Then one day, Frank had one of his practical ideas.

I loved writing letters, and was finding that holding a pen was becoming impossible. After only a few lines, I would go and run the hot water tap on my hands to ease the pain, and my writing was becoming quite illegible.

'I wonder if a typewriter would help?' asked Frank, out of the blue one Saturday morning.

So we got out the car, and drove to Watford, and bought a second-hand one, a great ugly office type necessitating two strong men to lift it on to the table.

It cost all of £2. 10s.

Now, I am not a great believer in miracles, or indeed of an Unseen Presence guiding one, but the first time I sat down at that typewriter, something wonderful did happen.

I had been a civil servant before my marriage. Not the secretarial kind, but one who filled in forms in triplicate, and used an adding-machine, but I had attended a short course of private typing lessons.

It was a school run by two sisters, the Misses Hay-thornthwaite, a couple of maiden ladies who smelled of rice-pudding, and still wore their hair in little plaited whorls over their ears.

They used a ruler to tap their pupils' wrists if the appropriate keys weren't tapped, and I had never forgotten the skill.

Typing is like riding a bicycle, or swimming; it is an accomplishment one never forgets, and although I was no longer a 'touch typist', at least four of my fingers being now out of action, I found I could still type at speed.

And as my swollen hands skimmed over the keys, I felt a moment of sheer elation. This was something I *could* do. This was me. . . .

So I wrote long letters to all my friends, friends who

111

must have been startled at ever hearing from me again, and when I'd practically worked my way through my address book, I just sat there, wondering vaguely if I couldn't prove myself by addressing envelopes, or better still, by typing the manuscripts of some local author.

Then a friend, one of the recipients of my typed letters, wrote back, and said she had read my letter aloud to her husband, who had actually laughed out loud – something of an occasion, according to her.

'Why don't you write stories?' she went on. 'I'm sure you could.'

I allowed the exciting thought to walk around in my mind for a few days. After all, I had mentioned it before, only to be told that I hadn't *lived* enough to write.

Then I remembered how Louisa M. Alcott had only succeeded when she had stopped writing adventure stories and concentrated on things she knew . . . her own family and their day to day experiences of life.

'I was always top of the class in Composition,' I told Frank that evening. 'I wrote about wanting to be a snowdrop when I was only seven, and I had to read it out to the whole school in Assembly.

'Why on earth should anyone in their right mind want to be a snowdrop?' asked Frank, and if I'd been the cushion-throwing type, I'd have thrown one at him there and then.

'You always liked the stories I told you about Claude the Centipede who had chilblains, didn't you?' I asked Marilyn, and she smiled at me with tolerance. She was, at that time, deeply in love with the boy who weighed out the potatoes at the greengrocer's, and inclined to treat my every remark with ill-concealed disdain.

'You could wear corduroy trousers and a beret, and type all day in the attic,' said Kate.

'And you can't spell,' said Frank.

But, ignoring them, I sat down at my beloved type-writer, the week before my fortieth birthday, and with a pan of soup simmering on the cooker, and the washing machine well into its third cycle, I wrote my first story.

Not knowing a thing about presentation, I typed it out in single spacing, on foolscap paper, a story about a mother going into hospital and leaving her young children behind. It was written with feeling, because of course it was the truth, a lavishly embroidered truth nonetheless, and it sold to the first magazine I sent it to. They wrote back and asked for more, and wanted to know would I accept £8 in payment?

Would I accept £8!

I wrote back graciously, and said I would, and then sat back and waited for the cheque to arrive. Because my knees were painful again, I got out my bicycle, and rode down to the bank to cash it when it arrived, and feeling like Lady Bountiful on one of her more generous days, distributed it amongst the four of us.

Two pounds each, I told them, to spend exactly as we liked. It was the first money I had earned since my marriage, and no money has ever been spent so joyously, or with such abandon.

Marilyn bought a petticoat, so stiff and voluminous that she had to come through the door sideways, Kate just wasted hers, Frank bought himself a magnificent paint-brush, and I treated myself to a bottle of bath oil, ensuring the softness of my skin for weeks to come.

There would be plenty more cheques to follow, I told my admiring family, and dashed off a couple of flippant love stories, only to have them returned in indecent haste by the editors of the magazines I'd sent them to.

But nothing could stop me now, and I realized that writing, like any other craft, has to be learned, so I started buying magazines, and studying the fiction, really studying it, as to style, theme, length, subject matter – the only way to succeed, I was convinced.

And whilst I was doing this, I wrote a book for children, which Nelsons published, not about Claude the Centipede, but about Kate's friendship with Peggy, a young American girl, whose parents had rented the house next door.

I was on my way . . . .

I didn't have time to think about my painful knees, ankles, wrists, and shoulders. I had read in a medical book that falling in love, going religious, or finding a new hobby were all good for the alleviation of swollen joints, and I reckoned that my method was as innocuous as any!

I started to do a correspondence course on the art of creative writing, and found that it taught me discipline, the necessary discipline if one is working at home, but I soon realized that writing is a flair, a gift, and can't be taught, and in my case I felt it to be a gift straight from the God I'd sometimes found it hard to believe in.

Everything that happened to me was grist to my mill, even my two week's stay in hospital for an ear operation provided a thoughtful little story for a woman's magazine, and a humorous one for radio's Morning Story.

Kind friends had told me that I would have to have my head shaved, so with the proceeds of my writing I went out and bought myself a wildly expensive wig.

Distorted hands, flat feet, and even three false teeth I could come to terms with, but not a bald head, and the first thing I did when I went into hospital was to set the wig up on its stand on my locker, giving Night Sister a nasty turn when she came round that first night.

It was dark, wavy and glamorous, and I felt like Elizabeth Taylor with wrinkles when I wore it, but the expense proved to have been unjustified when a little man approached my bed an hour before I was to go down to theatre, and draping me in a towel, proceeded to remove a few strands of hair from behind my right ear, and that was all.

Not long after her eighteenth birthday, Marilyn became engaged to a boy who lived just down the road, a boy I couldn't have liked better if I'd knitted him from a pattern I'd made myself, and Kate joined the Youth Club and brought home a boy who wrote poems, and took to walking down to the village in her bare feet. . . .

Then one day, cycling down to the Post Office to get a manuscript in the post, I swerved to avoid a small boy who ran into the road, fell off, and broke my leg in two places.

The left leg, the one with the badly affected knee of course, and I found myself once again back in hospital.

# 11

When an arthritic breaks a limb, especially if she's an arthritic on cortisone, things called complications can occur.

When I'd had my ear operation, they'd given me a massive boost of the stuff to raise my blood pressure which had dropped to a dangerously low level. My intake of the drug had already been cut down, and I wanted to be rid of the so-called miracle drug, yet now, tut-tutting over my broken leg, the doctors decided that I'd have to have a booster dose once again.

A miracle drug it may be, but once hooked on it, it seems there's no escaping from it.

Because the knee was badly affected by arthritis I was kept in plaster for only four weeks, and for eight more hobbled around the house on specially adapted crutches with shelves for my hands, being careful never to allow my bad leg to touch the ground.

I became adept at going upstairs backwards on my bottom, and sliding down by the same method with my injured leg outstretched, to the horror of anyone who happened to be present. With the help of my Friday lady I managed to get through the housework and cooking, hopping from the cooker to the fridge, my manipulated right ankle standing up bravely to the test. If only I'd known the trouble I was storing up for myself, I wouldn't have made such a game of showing off my one-legged prowess to anyone who dropped in.

We left the backdoor on the latch, and my friends made a rota to take it in turns to call, sitting around drinking coffee and smoking, and telling me how lucky I was not to have to go out in such filthy weather.

During those twelve weeks I could have written a longer book than *War and Peace*, but instead I sat and stared at the wall, in between hopping from one chore to another. Needless to say, when I did start writing again the first thing my heroine did was to go and break her leg!

Frank gave away my trusted bicycle, telling me that my cycling days were over, and I became a prisoner once more. But with a difference. My Lancashire grandmother would have said that my writing had taken me out of myself. Now I was earning money and could take taxis on the days I wasn't able to walk very far.

This was wonderful, but to this day I never pick up the telephone and call a taxi without experiencing the most enormous feelings of guilt. I'd been brought up to believe that taxis were for weddings, funerals and dire emergencies, and to take one to the shops or to visit a friend seemed so extravagant as to be almost indecent. I know I tend to overtip too, but this is because I want everyone, including taxi-drivers, to love me, so insecure am I.

These were my days of wine and roses, when I joined societies and made many writing friends. I would stand about at literary cocktail parties, balancing a glass in one hand and a triangular piece of toast topped with the tail end of an anchovy in the other, knowing that I'd pay for it the next day, and not giving a damn.

My nice kind doctor, convinced that the excitement of my new career was responsible for the improvement of my condition, took me off cortisone for good, and I tried the first of many anti-inflammatory drugs, each one heralded by the press as a miracle cure.

Marilyn got married, and I wore a red hat, the price of which I shall carry with me as a secret to my grave. A friend took a ciné film of the guests walking down the path from the church, and I am seen to be limping badly.

The red hat looks gorgeous, and it doesn't need the expertise of a lip-reader to see that I am confiding the fact to the bridegroom's father that my feet are killing me!

We turned Marilyn's bedroom into a study, lining the walls with my beloved books, and installing an extra telephone to tone with the new blue-grey carpet. Or was it the other way round?

I was finding it difficult to type, the pounding of the keys making my wrists swell so that I had to stop every so often to run the hot tap over my hands. The hospital occupational therapy department fashioned splints for me to wear as I typed, but I couldn't manage the buckles and straps and discarded them after a long struggle.

It began to look as if my typing days were over.

Then a friend lent me a tape-recorder. 'You just speak your stories into it, then get someone to type them out for you,' she said.

I am filled with admiration for writers who can work this way, especially those who can dictate their work to a secretary, but I was hopeless at it. My mind went completely blank, and then, when I forced myself to say a sentence, I was overcome with embarrassment, and found myself adopting the silly voice one uses to a telephone answering system.

So one day we drove into town and bought an electric typewriter. It solved my problem beautifully as it needs no pressure on the keys and has a carriage which slides along at a touch. Just one more blessing to count. . . .

Perhaps because I now considered myself artistic by nature, and slightly Bohemian to boot, I persuaded Frank to eat nuts and grated carrot with me at a health farm for a week. I was having trouble in sitting with any degree of comfort, a complication due to the bent knee.

I had been attending the hospital for weeks, having heat treatment, exercises, and spending a small fortune on taxi fares, all to no avail. So my gratitude knew no bounds when the osteopath at the health farm literally and painfully nipped the twisted nerve better for me. An osteopath works on the system that structural derangement of the body is the chief cause of disease. Their method is to adjust the affected parts by finger manipulation, and to leave the rest to nature.

It is a known fact that many rheumatologists think the day long overdue when osteopaths are included as a necessary part of their team in the big hospitals, but it is still true that many doctors still consider the majority of them to be mere quacks.

There, at the health farm, I was steamed, sweated, and rested, just as I had been steamed, sweated, and rested in the specialist hospital years ago.

We came home slim, bright-eyed and full of vitamin C, the result of all that fruit juice, and I couldn't wait to sit down at my typewriter and switch it on. There was a story that had to be written about a girl who went to a health farm. . . . She wouldn't have arthritis of course; her ambition would be to slim away the surplus pounds that were coming between her and romance. . . .

Marilyn's husband was sent out to Geneva for three years, and when their first baby was born, I flew out to her. A white-clad nun placed the baby in my arms as I stood on the balcony of a nursing home on the shores of Lake Léman, and I experienced one of those rare and precious moments of sheer joy. I was going to enjoy being a grandmother. I made a telephone call to Frank, describing the baby in lyrical terms, and he said he didn't mind being a grandfather. What he couldn't come to terms with was being married to a grandmother!

I felt I had so many blessings to count, surely arthritis was something I could shrug away, but changing nappies proved almost too much for me, and I knew that my support was more mental than physical. Something else would have to be tried, but what?

So once again we went in search of a cure, this time with the money earned by my writing burning a hole in my pocket. I was prepared to try anything.

So to Harley Street I went, to visit a doctor who specialized in diets. He maintained that we are what we eat, and that almost any complaint can be cured by eating the right foods.

It has been proved that three-quarters of the victims of rheumatoid arthritis go at one time or another for unorthodox healing. It is a great temptation, because honest medical men will not promise a cure.

This man, in all good faith, and with great sincerity, told me I must go on a diet which excluded meat, milk, acid fruits, fish, cheese, and anything not compost grown. In short any kind of food which tasted good. He was so handsome, so positively rude with health, so tanned, he would have made Tarzan himself appear to be suffering from anaemia. I was most impressed.

So, for a whole week I conscientiously ground nuts, steamed vegetables, drank plant milk which tasted, incidentally, like flour paste, and grated endless carrots. I cooked for Frank as usual, but told him that what he was eating was poison to his system and leading him to an early grave.

I aggravated him so much that one evening he took me out to the local restaurant and sat me down facing a large T-bone steak flanked on either side by glistening, salty chips.

I'd rather have you fat, limping and happy, than thin, hungry and fleet of foot,' he said, and who was I to argue with that?

The shopping centre was now way out of my range, so we invested in a deep-freeze cabinet, and after a few weeks of frantically trying to hack apart steaks frozen into a solid hunk five minutes before they were due to go underneath the grill, I learnt to get them out during the day, allowing them to thaw in their own good time.

Kate left school, did a course in journalism, and went up to Scotland to work on a magazine, meeting the boy up there she was to marry, another grand lad I couldn't

120

have loved more if I'd knitted him from my own pattern, and Marilyn, now back in England, added another Kathryn to the family.

So many good things were happening, there was so much to do, so many stories to write, friends to meet and talk shop to, I hadn't *time* to have arthritis. But all the time I knew that I was becoming more and more im- mobile, though I stubbornly refused to acknowledge it, even to myself.

Pollyanna worked extra hard for me during those years. . . .

I became interested in faith healing. I read a book which told me I could *will* myself back to health; I made notes from it and talked sternly to myself, but on Kate's wedding day I limped down the aisle to my place in the front pew, with the shuffling gait of a woman of 104.

Someone told me about acupuncture, and I made an appointment to see a practitioner who stuck needles in my right shoulder and my left knee. Although I was impressed, I had no relief from the arthritis, but believe that this form of treatment, like every other, works for some and not at all for others.

We didn't stagnate, however. Those were the years we flew abroad for holidays, to Yugoslavia, Portugal, Switzerland, and Austria, and I found that it was simpler for me to arrive at these faraway places than to get from my house to the shopping centre!

A car to the airport, transport to our hotel, and there I was, thousands of miles away, sitting on a balcony facing a foreign sea or a snow-capped mountain, sipping a glass of cognac, and counting my blessings like mad once again.

But oh, the ruins I would have liked to explore, the museums I wanted to visit, the narrow cobbled streets I would have loved to walk down, and that marvellous sun I would have given anything to lie in. Baking the joints is bad for arthritis, as so many doctors had told me over the years.

121

It was in Yugoslavia that I decided I was going to take up driving lessons, and this time I would make my arrangements before anyone could put a damper on them.

So the week after we returned home I rang an instructor and booked my first lesson.

He seemed delighted at the prospect of having me as a pupil, and before we said goodbye I said very quickly:

'There are one or two snags.'

There was the slightest of pauses.

'Yes, madam?'

'I would have to learn on an automatic car because my left leg is useless, and the wheel would have to have an adaptor on because of my hands, and I wouldn't be able to give hand signals, and I can't turn my head very far round, so reversing might be something of a problem.

The tone was rather subdued. 'Yes, madam.'

But I did have ten lessons and enjoyed every minute of them, and the instructor was a kind man who hinted that sometime in the far distant future I might even qualify to take a test. If he lived that long, his expression seemed to say as I put my good foot down hard on the accelerator pedal, getting speed up to all of twenty miles an hour.

Then, after using the handbrake my left wrist swelled up badly, and I had to realize that driving was not for me. And that was after ringing up a friend who lives in Birmingham and telling her that one fine day I'd be setting off and reaching her in a mere couple of hours.

Arthritis is a very mean complaint.

Kate was living with her husband up in Glasgow, and when she had a baby, our first grandson, I was put on the train and went to minister to her.

Again it was more moral support than anything. By now my daughters had completely reversed our positions. Now they cherished *me* instead of the other way round, and I wasn't sure whether I liked it or not. You see, in spite of the fact that I would be hard put to it to win a race with a half-doped tortoise, and in spite of the fact that when I look in the mirror a middle-aged face stares back at me, *inside* I am still seventeen, and a pretty nifty fleet-of-foot seventeen at that!

During the time I was in Glasgow, Kate gave me a good talking to.

'It's all very well accepting things, Mummy, but there are times when we have to fight.'

I laughed. 'And what do you think I've been doing all these years?'

And it was shortly after I came back home that surgery was mentioned to me for the first time, and I said I would consider it.

I went on considering it for the next few years, growing steadily more lame. Both girls lived within driving distance of me now, and two more babies were born, making five in all. It was touching to see how the children accepted me entirely as I was, climbing the stairs with me at a snail's pace, holding out little hands to help me up from a chair, playing a game of being Nannie as they limped up and down the hall with my stick.

Then, on one of my regular visits to the hospital, I was told in no uncertain terms that my knee joint, my shoulder, and my hands were so badly damaged that nothing short of surgery would help.

'A carpentry job,' the doctor said, and it seemed to make sense straight away.

Frank explained that if parts of his beloved car were worn out, he would have to replace them.

'And positive thoughts wouldn't help to replace brake-linings at all?' I said thoughtfully.

'Not at all,' said Frank.

'O.K., let's have a go,' I said, and it was arranged that I would meet the consultant of a big hospital specializing in joint operations.

So once again, Frank took a day of his leave and we set off on another journey of hope.

A lot of people tried to put me off the idea of surgery.

'They're only at the experimental stage, you know. You might find you're worse off than before,' said a friend, shaking her head sadly.

'But I could be better,' I said, and the friend said it was all wrong to tamper with nature.

'But nature has already tampered with me,' I said and changed the subject.

And as we drove to the hospital with Jimmy Young jollying us along on the car radio, I told myself that this was a chance I had to take; that slowly becoming a recluse was no answer, and that even an all-electric typewriter was no substitute for the company of friends, and the joys of a normal existence.

Again I submitted to examinations and X-rays, and the consultant, a tall young man with brilliantly blue eyes, explained in simple terms what they intended to do. It might have made sense to anyone with a practical turn of mind, but as far as I was concerned he could have been talking in a foreign language.

So Frank was called in to shake hands with yet another doctor in a white coat and to listen intently whilst the operation was spelt out to him in technical terms.

My own method of submitting to operations has always been to lie back, close my eyes, hold out my hand obligingly, and wait to be put to sleep. What goes on before I wake up again I'd rather be in ignorance of.

But Frank was fascinated. What the doctor was describing made sense to him because he is an engineer, and this time it was to be a reconstruction job. They were going to jack up the frayed edges of my knee joint, inserting a stainless-steel plate and doing what they called a synovectomy at the same time. The latter term means a scraping away of all the swollen and inflamed tissues.

I would have full movement again, because I had still retained a reasonable amount of mobility in the joint, and most important of all, I would be free from the excruciating pain. They stressed that if this initial operation didn't work, they would try another method, not wanting to do more than was absolutely necessary at first.

They talked about an operation on my hands, and explained that this entailed breaking the knuckles and inserting plastic pins, which would move as my fingers moved, and straighten the ever increasing slope. An operation on my shoulder wasn't advised as I had proved I could brush my hair and apply make-up with my left hand.

The consultant was so calm, so matter of fact, it was exactly as if he was telling a car owner what jobs needed doing to put his car back on the road again. . . .

'I'll be a new woman,' I told Frank as he turned the car out of the gates of the big hospital and out on to the main road again.

But Frank was driving slowly, inclining his head to listen for a mythical noise in the engine. He asked me to listen too, and for the next few miles we concentrated, until he decided it was merely my shortie umbrella rolling around on the back shelf.

Then he told me not to get excited about the forth-coming operation, and to take things in my stride, as I always did.

But being the way I am, I couldn't, and I stared unseeingly through the windscreen, not noticing the sudden spatter of raindrops. Awkwardly I leaned forward, and with my left hand, switched on the radio.

'Somewhere, over the rainbow,' sang Judy Garland in her catch-in-the-throat voice.

And it just *had* to be symbolic, I told myself.

# 12

This time, being a seasoned veteran, I prepared for my stay in hospital with as much attention to detail as a general preparing to do battle.

I bought a new face flannel, a flowing dressing-gown which would have more befitted the Hostess with the Mostest at a cocktail party, and enough deodorants and spray perfumes to ensure that come what might, I would always be nice to know.

We drove out to the freezer store and, leaning heavily on the wire trolley, I stocked up with enough frozen foods to keep not only Frank well nourished, but twenty-five friends should they choose to move in with him. With due regard to his aversion to cooking, I by-passed the wildly expensive joints of beef and lamb and concentrated on massive packs of hamburgers, and fish fingers, spending hours in the kitchen cooking casseroles in little silver foil dishes, telling him they only needed heating up.

That they were still there, frozen solid, when I came home didn't surprise me in the least.

I reminded Frank to leave the dustbin out on Wednesdays, the key in the porch for my Friday lady, and told him that if he used the electric blanket, not to forget to switch it off before he left for work each morning.

Settled into my hospital bed, I assured the house doctor that I didn't suffer from headaches, dizzy spells, ringing in the ears, chest trouble, heart palpitations, difficulty in passing water, hot flushes, indigestion, allergies or double vision. I felt it was the least I could do, especially as what I was forced to tell her covered three foolscap pages!

That first day I was given an ice-pack to drape over my swollen knee, and another for my wrist, which had produced a lump as big as a ducks' egg, perhaps to justify my being there!

So much for the soaking in hot water, and the many hours basking in the warmth of my infra-red lamp.

'Heat only makes the inflammation worse. Ice contracts the tissues and reduces the swelling,' I was told.

Tests and more tests, and a session with the occupational therapist to demonstrate how I turned on taps, filled a kettle, coped with screw-topped jars, and picked up scattered pins.

'What about zips?' she asked me, and I told her that I managed with a hook gadget at the end of a long cord, but that if I mislaid it, which was every other day, I had either to arrive with my dress undone at the back, or call upon anyone handy to help. The milkman, the taxi-driver, the man calling to read the meter, even the curate, have all zipped me up on occasions. . . .

The evening before the operation, a small contingent of doctors and surgeons came round the ward. One of them drew black arrows on my knee, and Sister explained that I would wake up in the recovery ward, where I would spend twenty-four hours in strict isolation as a protection against infection. Then, just half an hour later, the house doctor came and told me that a report had come from the laboratory showing that I had a slight urinary infection, and that they daren't operate. I was to go home and be re-admitted two weeks later after a course of antibiotic tablets which would clear up the trouble.

I am not given to outward demonstrations of feelings, totally incapable of floods of tears, but it was like climbing the guillotine and laying a head on the block, only to be told to come back the next day because the knife wasn't sharp enough, and for a moment I could only

127

stare at him in disbelief.

I rang Frank and he came for me, and I rang the girls and thanked them for the lovely flowers I'd had to leave behind, and we got the marks off my knee with turpentine.

I swallowed the tablets dutifully, and wrote a story about a girl who had been jilted at the altar. Freud could have explained the working of my mind quite clearly, I'm sure.

Then once again I packed my little bag, but this time I didn't say goodbye to anyone. Like the Arabs, I'd decided, I would silently slip away. . . .

So, at long last, attired in a little white shift, plus matching turban and knickers, my wedding ring covered with tape, and my shame-making dental-plate in a plastic dish, I was wheeled to the theatre.

My first thought when I came to in the recovery ward was blessed relief that it was all over, my second was to ask for my denture, and my third was one of total disbelief.

Surely the patient in the opposite bed wasn't a MAN? Through a drowsy mist of ether I ascertained that if it was a woman, then she had long side-burns and a droopy moustache, then I lay back on my pillows and realized that unisex was everywhere, even in hospital.

Half of an enormous bandage covering my knee was removed after one week, and a week after that, the stitches were removed, quite painlessly. The scar was no more than six inches long, the swelling had completely gone, and I found I could lift my leg straight up and even bend it slightly. I showed it proudly to all my visitors, and only Jamie, my little grandson, seemed disappointed that there wasn't more blood about.

'He was sure they were going to cut your leg off,' his mother told me, and I said I was sorry to have let him down.

It wouldn't be true to say that when I tried to walk I felt no pain. My ankles had rebelled against their enforced rest in bed, and as I tottered that first day to the dining-room on crutches, sweating and aching with the effort, I wished with all my heart and very soul that they'd left me as I was. An arthritic knee I had come to terms with, but a steel plate was another matter.

But each day showed a slight improvement, and when I was home I was able to discard the crutches and get around the house with one stick. My knee was knee-shaped once again, and the six-inch scar was already beginning to fade, but I found going up and down stairs a sweating, arduous procedure.

'You ought to live in a bungalow,' a friend scolded, 'certainly not in a house without a downstairs loo.'

'If we lived in a bungalow, I would lose the ability to climb stairs, and the world outside is full of stairs,' I said, and my friend said she despaired of me.

Before she left she took a cutting from the local paper out of her handbag and placed it on the hall table.

'Pride can be a very over-rated emotion,' she told me as she said goodbye. 'Why don't you ring that number one of these days? I'm sure there are lots of ways in which you could be helped.'

I closed the door behind her and picked up the news-paper cutting.

**IF YOU NEED HELP**, it said in large black capitals, then went on to give a list of telephone numbers. SOME SERVICES AVAILABLE AS OF RIGHT TO ELDERLY AND HANDICAPPED PEOPLE, it went on.

I stood there for a long time, actually tracing the appropriate number with my finger, then I opened the little cupboard which houses the directories, and push-ing it inside, firmly closed the door. I wasn't ready to stretch out a hand yet. . . .

But we didn't book a holiday abroad that year. Instead we drove down to South Devon, staying at a small hotel perched atop a wooded cliff, with a magnificent view of the bay dotted with tiny ships, their orange sails vivid in the sunshine. Because of the steep gradient which made it almost impossible for me to take as much as a single step outside, I spent hours sitting on the terrace communing with Mother Nature, whilst Frank closeted himself in the television room, communing equally happily with the World Cup, and tennis from Wimbledon.

It was on my third day that I discovered a shame-making truth about myself. Views bored me rigid!

I tried, I honestly did. I stared at all those trees with their leafy mouths pressed like mad against the earth's sweet flowing breast, and I told myself for good measure that only God could have made them, and it didn't do a thing for me.

Whilst everyone else was going on about the curling mist creeping over the horizon, and the way those dear little boats were pure poetry, I was sitting there wondering why that fat woman had chosen to wear a jumper with the stripes going round her enormous bosom, and trying to fathom what that gorgeous young girl could possibly see in that middle-aged balding little man.

It doesn't help me as a writer either. . . .

Think what a help it would be to me if I could describe the way the buttercups sang to each other in the meadow, and the way a tiny leaf could fill my heroine's heart with pure and unbounded joy in the mystery of creation.

But then, I can honestly say I've never in the whole of my life heard a buttercup sing, and russet leaves on the ground just remind me to watch my step even more than usual.

'I could sit here for ever,' a lady in a turquoise anorak told me one morning, feasting her eyes on the rain belting down and wetting all those trees. 'I swear I can smell the grass growing.'

That was when I went up to my room to make myself a cup of coffee with the electric kettle thoughtfully provided by the management, and there I read a magazine

130

story about an elderly hippie who fell in love with the chairman of the Women's Institute, and changed her life for the better.

Now *he* didn't waste his time going around smelling the grass growing, for goodness' sake!

'Just look at that view,' Frank said, coming into the room and catching me with my back to it.

I said I'd seen it hadn't I, and it looked just the same when it was raining, except that it was wet. . . .

Maud might have been persuaded to go out into the garden where the black bat night had flown, I told him, but I was perfectly all right where I was, without a leafy bud in sight.

I was fortunate that I'd never been one for the Great Outdoors, because in spite of the plate in my knee I was finding it increasingly difficult to get around. Surgery is fine, but obviously it only helps the joint concerned. Now my feet and ankles were rebelling, and I was forced to give up my trips to town. I could no longer walk to the shops, even if I sat for a while in the library to recover, enjoying a free read of *Vogue* and the *Financial Times*. I put my immobility down to the humidity and told the doctor in yet another hospital which was only a five minutes' taxi ride away that come winter I would improve.

He told me about a club he was hoping to organize, run by, and for, arthritic patients of the hospital, an ambitious venture in which sufferers were to be taught to understand the complexities of their complaint, and in so doing learn to cope with the difficulties.

Its aims were to be widespread and varied, ranging from an increased knowledge of all rheumatic disorders, to the practical self-help and outside support which is available to patients. Talks would include such topics as the availability of Social Services, orthopaedic surgery, exercises and the reason for them, and the various treatments now in current use in the fight against the disease.

I promised to go along to the first meeting as a member

131

of what was to be an inner committee, and because I mentioned that I could type, found myself being nominated as Secretary.

'It's a kind of Arthritics Anonymous,' I told Frank after the meeting.

'And you're keen on the idea?'

We were sitting round the television, watching it with the sound turned down as we often do, to enable us to carry on a conversation.

'Why do you sound so doubtful?' I asked him, and he got his pipe going nicely before he replied.

'Because you've always said that you wished to avoid the company of people afflicted in the way you are – that swapping symptoms is definitely not your thing.'

There was a beautiful young girl on the television screen agonizing soundlessly over something or other, but we ignored her.

'You mean that bit about me not thinking about myself as an arthritic, but as an ordinary woman who just happens to have arthritis?'

Frank nodded.

I sat still for a while without speaking. It was what they call in fiction the Moment of Truth. Then I turned my back on my mental Pollyanna for the first time in almost thirty years, and *spoke* the truth.

'I *am* an arthritic, and more than that, I'm a disabled person,' I said straight out. 'Tonight I realized it somehow. I saw women who need help, the help this new club will give, and I need help, and mustn't be too proud to ask for it.'

I was being dramatic, and I knew it, but I couldn't help myself. I am sure that in everyone who writes there's a little demon, silently cheering them on from the wings.

'I *am* disabled,' I said again.

Frank just nodded. 'Now we can do something about it, love, and I suggest that the first thing in the morning you get out that newspaper cutting you've hidden in the hall cupboard, and ring that number. O.K.?'

132

'Have I been impossible?' I asked him quietly.

He shook his head. 'No, not impossible. Just too blasted stubborn for words,' he said, but he was smiling at me.

The voice when I dialled the number was young and sympathetic. When she said 'Can I help you?' it sounded as if she really meant it. I could sense her waiting patiently as I stumbled over the words which should have been so easy to say.

I was trying hard not to resort to flippancy, but a life-time's habit dies hard, so I told her that I'd heard that if a person was registered as disabled, then that person could have a sticker for the car, giving the driver certain advantages whilst parking.

'I went shopping with my husband last Saturday, and the car park was so far from the shops I had to sit in the car and wait for him. And he hates shopping,' I said, truthfully.

'Are you registered as a disabled person?' the girl listening to me asked.

This was it.

'No, but I think I should be,' I said.

The following week a small yellow car drew up in the road outside, and a young girl wearing trousers and a scarlet top, with her short dark hair framing her pretty face, rang the doorbell.

I'm your Disabled Living Adviser,' she said, and smiled at me, and she was so much like my own two daughters that it would have been impossible for me not to feel at ease with her.

In that first short visit, without seeming to have noticed anything, she arranged for me to be registered, a perfectly painless procedure. She told me I would be given a disc which fastened to the windscreen of the car, and would make life much easier for me.

She asked to see the bathroom, and I told her that I had long given up the luxury of lying down in the water, and had been forced to take far less satisfying showers.

She cast an expert eye over the height of the lavatory seat, and came a few days later with a loose throne-like seat, which made my legs dangle, but also made getting on and off much simpler. She brought a straight board which fitted over the bath, enabling me to swing my legs over, and a seat which meant that at least part of me could be submerged in water.

She arranged for handles to be fixed to walls at strategic places, and in due course a pleasant man with a face like a contour map of Ireland came and screwed chrome-plated handles to the tiles in the bathroom, and a rail to the wall at the top of the stairs, and departed assuring me that he would be sure to Jaysus to remember me in his prayers.

It was impossible, it seemed, to have a downstairs loo built in. Two men from the Social Services came and measured and shook their heads, but they asked me how I would feel about having a lift installed, if this proposition was passed by the Council – a platform-like contraption fixed to the wall side of the staircase, which would move up and down at the touch of a switch.

They even arranged for me to go and see a man who lived locally who had had one put in, and so off we went, and Frank and I rode solemnly up and down this nice stranger's staircase. We then drank sherry with him, a widower who lived all alone with the memories of his wife, in a room hung with her paintings, vivid Spanish scenes glowing brightly against dull green walls.

I was given brochures so that I might study the right kind of high chair to buy, and advised to drop hints to Father Christmas about an electric carving knife, so that the slicing of meat and bread would be less of a strain.

So much kindness, so much concern, all given at a time when our National Health Service was under so much criticism. When all the country seemed to be under the impression that it was Number One that counted, and that selfishness and unconcern were the order of the day.

And all because I lifted the telephone receiver one day. . . .

So what has it taught me? After almost thirty years of trying to go it alone? Of kidding myself that I was different, that I needed and would accept help from no one?

I admit now that there is, at the present time, no cure for arthritis. I know that it is Britain's most widespread disease. More people have it than any other complaint, and only one person in fifty will escape some form of it by the time they reach the age of seventy.

And two-thirds of these are women.

It is not caused by the wearing out of the joints, but by some unknown agency which research is trying to track down. The cost to the nation is approximately £225,000,000 per annum in lost wages alone, without the cost of treatment, hospital beds and drugs. The true cost will run in thousand of millions of pounds every year.

On the brighter side, there is a strong feeling among researchers that soon the breakthrough will come, and knowing the cause, they will be able to provide the antidote for arthritis.

Till that day comes, it is for me, and countless thousands like me, back to the aspirins, the gold injections, the drugs, the positive thoughts, the counting of blessings, and the hope that one day, in some laboratory, the long and dedicated search for a cure will be rewarded.

# 13

It was a whole year afterwards before I admitted that the operation to insert a plate into my knee joint hadn't done what the doctors hoped it would do. I was limping badly, and the consultant at the vast new hospital was not to be taken in by any display of feminine heroics.

He was straightforward, kind and honest, and he had the type of face to which one told the truth and nothing but the truth, and besides, I was feeling so ill that I actually admitted it.

I ought to have known better. From past experience I should have known that before long I would find myself back in bed, in a corner of some ward or other.

But now, for some reason, I had learnt to cry again. My tear-ducts, which had been dammed for so many years, had opened up again.

Whereas before I could listen, apparently unmoved, to the most harrowing details of suffering, even of death itself, dry-eyed and composed, now I could cry with abandon.

I found myself sobbing through each weekly instalment of *This is Your Life* on television, long before the subject's long-lost brother had been specially flown from Australia. And only the week before my visit to the hospital, I'd cried my eyes into fiery slits all through the quite innocuous rendering of the Hallelujah Chorus sung by a massed choir, relayed from the Albert Hall.

So when I told about my recent symptoms, especially the agonizing pain spreading from the back of my neck into my head, the shameful tears were already pricking away behind my eyelids.

Therefore I ought not to have been surprised when the consultant reached for the telephone on his desk.

'I think we'll have your wife in for an assessment,' he told Frank who had taken a day of his leave to help me keep the appointment.

'For how long?' I asked, the tears escaping now, and running in self-pitying rivulets down my cheeks.

'One or two weeks,' said the doctor vaguely, and it was like a record being played over again, one we had heard so often we should have heard it without the slightest flinch.

'At least *this* hospital is on my way home from work,' said Frank, 'I can call in to see you on my way home.

'Two weeks will soon pass,' I said.

'Just get yourself put right,' said Frank, as he had so often said before, and the next day I pulled the black cover over my beloved typewriter, took a last glance round my little room, and climbed into the car for the short drive to the hospital.

'I'll kiss you goodbye here in the car,' said Frank, knowing my dislike of demonstrations of affection in public, so solemnly we kissed. He helped me out of the front passenger seat, got my case out of the boot, and together we walked through the big glass doors into the wide reception area.

It was 8.30 on a Saturday evening, a time when most young men are out for a drink with their friends. A time for taking a girlfriend out to dinner, or merely sitting back in a chair with a can of beer on the arm, listening to records. But the young doctor who came to my bed, swishing the curtains round with a practised hand, was still working. He held the inevitable list of questions clipped to a board, and showed no sign of the tiredness he must have felt. He was 'bleeped' away to another ward before he was halfway through his examination, but he returned still smiling, apologizing for the delay.

At the end of an eighty-hour week, his take-home pay would, I knew, be less than many manual workers are paid for forty hours' work, but he listened carefully to my replies, actually laughing out loud now and again when I said something that amused him.

His examination took a long time, and after he'd gone on his way, white coat flying, I lay down and stared into the darkened ward, and tried to remember if I'd told Frank about the sponge cake in the tin that needed eating up before its layer of cream went off. . . .

There were four beds in the ward, and once again I was thrust into sharing an intimate relationship with perfect strangers. Two of the women were arthritics, I knew that because they'd told me before the young doctor came, but the other bed was occupied by a ravishingly pretty young woman with hair so fair that it actually appeared to glitter. She had the type of looks that James Bond seems to prefer, all sweeping eyelashes and pouting lips, but intelligent with it, and I could see that she was reading a magazine in the light that came from the corridor outside.

Of late, instead of counting sheep – their silly faces had always irritated me anyway – I had taken to saying the Twenty-third Psalm over to myself when I couldn't go to sleep. It had a warm and soothing effect, and stopped me from turning endlessly trying to find a comfortable position.

'Yea, though I walk through the valley of the shadow of death,' I silently intoned, and then I thought about all the patients in that vast hospital who *were* perhaps walking through the valley, maybe at that *very* moment. . . . It was too much for me, and I reached for a tissue and pulled the sheet over my head.

The next morning I was fascinated to see the James Bond girl sit up in bed and fix her false eyelashes into position before the early cup of tea came round. She wore a lace nightie with a neckline cut to advantage, and I never did find out what was wrong with her because she went home that day, collected by a husband who was as beautiful as she was. Whatever was wrong with her didn't *show*, that much was certain. . .

Her bed was immediately claimed by a big man with grey sideboards and a stomach which rested on his knees when he sat down.

'I don't mind being in here with the ladies, ducks,' he told Sister, 'they're safe enough with me, worse luck.' And the stomach wobbled as if it had a separate life of its own.

But unisex hadn't gone quite that far, and there was a shuffle round of beds. I was given a small side-ward with a single bed in it. I was thrilled. I saw myself sitting there typing away like mad, or even lying there with the type-writer balanced on my chest, emerging at the end of my two week' stay with the first draft of a novel tucked away beneath my nighties with their matching bed-jackets.

The fact that I can't manage to use any typewriter that isn't electrically driven, and that the weight of one on my chest would stop my breathing in five minutes flat didn't seem to matter. I was quite carried away by the thought of being alone in that tiny room.

I get exactly the same feeling when I close the door of my small study at home, and once I tried to explain this to a friend.

'Back to the womb, dear,' she said, which was very clever of her. I would never have thought of a reason like that, not in a million years. I just thought I liked being alone at times. . . .

So there I was, imagining the little side-ward filled to overflowing with friends at visiting time. They would crowd round my bed and drink my health in Lucozade, and tell me how nasty it was outside, and how awful the news was, and how lucky I was not to be braving the one or listening to the other.

My grandchildren would come, all five of them – gone were the days when children were not admitted on visit-ing days, in this enlightened hospital anyway – and Lucy, who climbs on everything, would sit there on my bed, and Daniel who once kissed a Father Christmas smack in the middle of his rather scruffy beard, would kiss all the nurses and enchant them. Jamie would ask pointed questions like when was I going to die, Kathryn would come and lean up against me for her customary cuddle, and Alison would open one of my magazines and be immediately lost to the world.

So overcome was I by my unexpected isolation that I almost forgot what I was in for, but an assessment was what they had said, and an assessment was what I was going to get!

Once more I was X-rayed.

'Now how can I have arthritis *there*?' I asked the coffe-coloured girl in charge of the massive machines as she took a photograph of my open mouth.

'Nothing at all to worry about, dear,' she told me with a gentle smile, and I said I didn't want to worry, I merely wanted to *know*. But she glided away from me, bearing my dental plate in a round dish, as if she knew that was the one way to stop me asking silly questions.

Why shouldn't a patient in hospital ask questions? That's something I've always wanted to know. I'd been asked the most intimate details about my bodily functions, and some rather pointed ones about my family too. In one hospital a young doctor had been so completely fascinated by my account of an attack of scarlet fever when I was nine years old that he'd quite forgotten what I was there for.

I determined to ask the consultant whether it was possible to have arthritis of the tonsils, but forgot all about it as apparently my blood tests and urine samples had been checked and I was to be given the opportunity of having gold injections.

Gold is one of the most ancient medicines known to man, and it was introduced as a treatment for arthritis in 1934. It has to be given by injections, having no effect at all if swallowed, and it is administered every week in small doses. It does help a great deal in a high percentage of cases, but it may take three or four months before any beneficial effects are noticed.

I knew that even after leaving the hospital I would still have to return week after week for the injections, and I knew also that it wouldn't cure my arthritis.

'But it's a golden opportunity,' I told Frank that evening, unable to resist the awful pun, then I told him that a surgeon was coming to see me the next day.

We stared at each other, whilst two invisible thought bubbles hovered over our heads:

'NOT ANOTHER OPERATION!' they said.

I was lying flat on my bed with one toe pointing in the vague direction of the ceiling when the surgeon walked into my room early the next morning.

I'd been given an illustrated list of daily maintenance exercises to do, each one designed to keep the muscles working. I was able to do only about one in three, but had promised to do them on first waking to overcome stiffness.

The list also advised a rest of one hour daily, preferably lying face down on the bed, with one or no pillows. It was very firm about the bad habit of lying with a painful knee supported by a cushion, and it reminded me again that knitting was *not* advisable.

The surgeon introduced himself, then examined my knee, prodding it gently with long clever fingers. He told me he had seen the X-ray, and that in his opinion, an operation to remove the plate and the worn-out parts of the joint, replacing them with artificial parts, would be the only thing that would help.

I listened to his quiet voice, trying hard to understand. I knew that I trusted him – he had a direct and honest way of expressing himself, and he made no promises, merely told me the facts.

'But wouldn't it improve with the passage of time? The gold injections I'm going to have? The exercises I'm going to do every day?' I felt I had to make a stand somehow.

He shook his head, and explained that the artificial joint would be made of steel and plastic, and would be lubricated by the body's natural secretions. He told me, pulling no punches, that this operation was of fairly recent origin, but they were hopeful about its durability. It was already known, he said, that artificial hip joints lasted for at least fifteen years.

'And the success rate of the knee job?' I felt bound to ask.

'Very good,' he assured me, the twinkle in his eyes preventing me from asking him to swear on his very life that this time it would work.

'When a joint is as badly destroyed as your knee, there is really no other way,' he said, then, in spite of the fact that every minute of his time was precious, he patiently drew me a little diagram showing exactly what he proposed to do.

'Think it over,' he said kindly as he left me, and I lay back, the exercises forgotten. As usual, before accepting quite passively what was to happen to me, I tortured myself by imagining the worst. . . .

There I was, just round from the anaesthetic, groping around beneath the sheet trying to find the twin to the one pathetic leg stretched out in front of me.

'Sorry, dear, but that's the way it goes sometimes,' they would tell me, and I stared down at my legs and actually wondered if it had been a waste of time to apply pink nail polish to both feet. I shuddered and picked up the exercise chart again, and as I rotated my elbows in a clockwise direction, I was counting, not the fifteen seconds advocated, but the hours until visiting time.

'Make up my mind for me,' I pleaded with Frank that evening.

'Show me a sign,' I asked God in my prayers that night.

But it was all up to me, and all I wanted to do was to go home and get on with my life. What was a limp anyway? And the pain? Well I was used to that by now, and if my mental Pollyana had as much as peeped at me from behind my locker, I'd have hit her straight between the eyes with the bunch of grapes rotting gently in my fruit dish.

If a nurse had come to take my temperature I'd have bitten off the end of the obnoxious little tube, and if anyone had told me I was a real tonic, I'd have spat right in their eye!

I might have earned a reputation as a good patient, but from now on, things were going to be different.

There'd be no more waking up obediently to take my sleeping tablet; no more sticking to my principle of ringing my bell for other patients only, and only then if they happened to have burst their stitches or had just turned blue.

Now, for some reason, I was good and mad, and mean with it too. Now, for the first time in all those years, I found myself asking, 'Why *me*?'

The feeling didn't last for long, but I revelled in it while it lasted. I left off my lipstick and the touch of blusher I use; I wore a once-yellow nightie which had turned a sickly fawn in the wash, and for good measure, instead of leaving out my morning specimen I flushed it triumphantly down the lavatory pan.

But it's quite true that a leopard never changes its spots, because when the consultant came on his round, accompanied by his retinue, I told him that I felt fine, and was pefectly happy – without a care in the world, I'd have gone on to say, if encouraged.

'Made up your mind?' he asked me, holding up the X-ray picture of my knee, and explaining to everyone that the damage to my joint was serious.

He asked me to get up and walk towards him, and I tried. I tried with all my will-power to put on a good performance, but it was no use.

Staggering like a drunken woman, I managed to pull myself to my feet by hanging onto a radiator, then I shuffled painfully towards him.

'I really have no choice, have I?' I said, and he smiled at me, shaking his head, but I knew that the decision must be mine alone.

'I'll have it done,' I said, and actually thanked him very much. . . .

The surgeon came to see me again that same day, and said that I would have to go home for a few weeks until he could fit me into his schedule, and I thanked him, too. Then I got dressed and packed my little case and imagined the look on Frank's face when I told him he could take me home with him that evening.

I wheeled the portable telephone into my room and talked to the girls, and they both said that it was for the best, that things usually turned out for the best; and a friend came that afternoon, and she said that it was for the best too.

Then at 4 o'clock a young lady doctor with brown curly hair came into my room and beamed at me from the foot of my bed.

'Great news!' she said. 'A patient who was to have surgery on Monday morning has gone home, so we can do you then. Isn't that splendid?'

'Absolutely marvellous,' I said still smiling like the hypocrite I am, but she was right of course. No time for second thoughts that way, no settling down into my routine of domesticity and writing, only to have it disrupted once again.

And within minutes I was whisked away in a wheelchair, my case on my knee, and a potted plant underneath my arm, down long corridors into a lift and down another corridor into the surgical ward.

The wheelchair seemed symbolic somehow. It had been taken for granted that I *needed* it, and the idea didn't appeal at all.

There were three other patients in my new ward, all arthritic cases. We very soon got down to swapping symptoms, all trying to outdo each other as to the amount of suffering we'd had over the years. One young woman, a victim of Still's disease, had had bones removed from the balls of her feet to make walking less painful, and wore contraptions extending from her toes which looked like harp strings.

Still's disease is a form of rheumatoid arthritis which affects very young children, often between the ages of one and three years. As in the adult version, early treatment is essential.

A bright-eyed little lady in the bed next to mine told me that she had had her hip 'done' only five months before, and that her knee joint had been replaced the previous week. Naturally I had more than a passing interest in her condition, and went over to talk to her.

Her leg was swollen to roughly four times its size by bandages which extended from her ankle to her thigh, but she assured me that if she didn't move it, she was in no pain at all.

What she didn't tell me was that already she was 'exercising' it, trying to lift it straight up, all part of the necessary after operation care, so when I was told I could go home for the weekend I felt reassured and told Frank that I was quite looking forward to the operation.

'No need to overdo it, love,' he said, as yet once again we trailed round the supermarket. He was so used to being left to cope on his own by now that I merely leaned on the wire trolley as he filled it up with 'whole meal' soups, and exotic sounding tins of prawns in jelly, and anything in fact that didn't need cooking.

I reported back at the appointed hour, and whilst Frank was sitting by my bed the anaesthetist came and explained to me, not realizing that I was a veteran, that I would have a calming injection before I went up to theatre early the next morning, and that he would be there, taking good care of me.

He was so gentle, so handsome in a David Niven kind of way, that I couldn't help flirting with him, much to Frank's amusement.

'If you wear dentures, they will have to be removed,' he told me, and I confided that in all the thirty-two years of our marriage, Frank had never seen me without my 'plate'.

'Don't speak to me when I'm toothless, because I won't answer you,' I teased, and he thought for a moment then said that he would arrange for me to keep them in, and he would remove them personally when I was unconscious.

That, in itself, was indicative of the utter kindness and understanding which was to be shown to me in the weeks to come. Of course I said that I wouldn't be so foolish, and when the time came I handed over my dentures quite happily to the nurse.

'They'll be right here on your locker, honey,' she said, as she helped me on with a white cotton shift with bikini briefs to tone.

She gave me my soothing injection, and I was so relaxed by the time I was wheeled up to theatre that I smiled a gummy smile at the anaesthetist, and after it was all over, vaguely remembered stroking his hand as he administered the knock-out injection.

'How kind you are, so nice, so lovely,' I murmured, and I hope but doubt it very much, that I made his day!

# 14

As the swallowing of half a sleeping tablet can send me into a death-like coma and render me capable of uttering words of one syllable only until three o'clock the next day, it wasn't surprising that the four weeks following the second operation to my knee passed in a hazy dream.

'It's the anaesthetic working itself gradually out through the pores after blocking up your whole system,' I was told by a patient in a blue quilted dressing-gown.

Her right hand was heavily bandaged after an operation to correct the sideways slope of her fingers, and I could see the way she was staring at my hands which at the time were folded idly over my chest.

'They'll be doing your hands next, I expect?' she said hopefully but kindly. 'Why don't you ask them if you can stay in and have everything done at one go?'

'Now there's a nice thought,' I said. I closed my eyes and was lost in a vision of myself jointless and covered in operation scars, every movable part of me replaced by gadgets made of steel and plastic.

I had been told, however, that as my hands were fairly functional, in spite of their deformity, the procedure was to leave well alone. Early surgery *can* be performed on hands not too badly affected, and this is called a synovectomy, but mine were too far gone for that, and an operation on them would involve a replacement of the knuckle joints.

I could still manage to dress myself, even if it was a struggle at times, and I could type, and not for the first time I wondered if my daily stint at my electric typewriter had kept my fingers mobile.

So I dismissed my gruesome thoughts, sat up in bed, and went on with what I'd been doing.

This consisted of staring into space, the books I'd bought in with me to improve my mind unopened, the jigsaw puzzles undone, and my 'thank you' letters unwritten. I was far more interested in eavesdropping on what the doctors were saying to the patient across from me, as I was absolutely fascinated by other patients' symptoms and willing to go on at length about my own.

I found myself sinking into a state of complete apathy, happy to become thoroughly institutionalized, not caring in the least that in the world outside there were strikes and famines, threats of wars, hi-jacks and murders, muggings and rapes.

Then at last the bandages were removed from my leg, the stitches neatly and painlessly removed from the long scar down the middle of my knee, and I hobbled round the ward on elbow crutches, specially designed for patients like me who can't manage the more orthodox kind.

There was a long corridor flanking the wards and I used this as my training ground, trying hard to remember to keep my head up, my tail tucked in, my legs straight, my eyes looking ahead, and my weight evenly balanced on both feet.

I was amazed and delighted to find that the pain in my knee was hardly worth mentioning, in fact my ankles were the culprits, but I put this down to the long rest in bed.

Now the exercises I'd learnt were all important, and day after day the physiotherapist, a very pretty young girl wearing the regulation white blouse and short red skirt, came and put us all through our motions. I was taught to press my knee down hard into the mattress, until I could actually see the muscle working, then to lift my leg up straight. This was to correct any 'lag' that may have developed.

Soon I graduated to two sticks, and when the time came to go home I was able to walk to the car in a more or less upright position.

The fact that my new knee would bend sufficiently for me to get into the car, pleased me no end, and I insisted on getting out and doing it again just to show off. I was equally thrilled to find that I could climb the stairs without pain, taking one step at a time and going very slowly, but getting there just the same.

'The first thing I'm going to tell the disablement officer when she calls is that I no longer need the lift,' I said, and it was agreed that instead I would have a bar fixed to the wall, parallel with the banister, a great help in coming down as I can only lift one arm.

But because of the longish walk to the shops I found that I was still virtually housebound during the day. With the help of one stick I would take short walks down the avenue, talking to cats on walls, and getting to know the houses so well I could have reproduced every single grain of pebble-dash.

For the first month at home I was allocated a home help, a bonny Irish woman who took over the running of my home for two hours twice a week as if she'd always been a friend of the family. She needed showing only once where the dusters and polishes were kept, and would leave me with a tidy house, Frank's shirt from the day before hanging out to dry, and a casserole prepared for the oven. My faithful cleaning lady came as usual on her Friday morning, so I was able to sit around with my leg stretched out on a stool.

Part of me was still back in the hospital. I still woke at six longing for the early cup of tea, and wished I could wash with a bowl of water on my bedside table, instead of getting up and walking the few steps into the bathroom. I found myself wondering how the patients I'd left behind were faring, and on my weekly visits for my gold injection, would make my way into the ward, catching up on their progress, and half resenting the new patient who was sitting up in *my* bed.

Because we found that getting up from our low chairs and sofa left me sweating and demoralized, we bought a special 'geriatric' chair, so high from the ground that my feet dangled when I sat in it. Getting up out of it was no problem at all, as I was more than halfway there already!

It meant that I could answer the door-bell before the person ringing it had given up in disgust and disappeared down the avenue, and I was glad of the chair, and yet hated it, just as I hated anything which stressed my disability.

The children loved it, however, and would fight for possession of it, taking turns at sitting there enthroned, monarchs of all they surveyed.

My lovely disablement officer explained how we could raise our own chairs and my bed on wooden blocks, and as we'd moved into the guest room with its twin beds, I was able to lie there, inches higher than Frank, tossing and turning to my heart's content.

We still slept in the double bed at weekends, however, remembering no doubt that both our Lancashire grandmothers had said that twin beds, as far as marriage went, were the 'beginning of the end.'

I became used to seeing Frank trotting uncomplainingly up and down the landing with our tea-making machine, making sure that it was in the right room at the right time. . . .

'The day you tell me you've started writing again, I'll know you're feeling better,' he said, but my mind was a formless blank. I told him that in all probability I'd never write again; that I couldn't think why I'd ever thought I could write anyway, and that I was going to teach myself to crochet as knitting was forbidden.

So there I sat, in my special chair, struggling with instructions that sounded Greek to me, trying to wind the wool round my knobbly fingers. The pattern I'd chosen said that a child of seven could do it. 'A child with an I.Q of 503!' I muttered underneath my breath.

My effort turned out as a sweaty, lumpy length of knotted wool, bearing so little resemblance to the neat shell-like edging in the illustration that I rolled it into a ball and hid it away underneath the table-mats in the sideboard drawer.

'Why don't you at least *try* to write a short story?' Frank asked me one day when I told him I'd spent my afternoon sticking Green Shield stamps in books, copying out recipes I knew I'd never try, and watching a film on television, the girlish leading lady of which was now retired and drawing her old age pension.

'Because every idea I get is trivial,' I said with a melancholy sigh. 'If I did start to write again it would have to be an in-depth piece about suffering and what is *real*. If I wrote anything at the moment it would make a pair of gloomy Chekhov characters sound as if they were a Music Hall turn.'

'Surely you're not getting *depressed*?' said Frank, amazed, but I just turned away and went on seeing the black side of everything and reading books telling me how to snap out of it, leaving me sadder than ever.

Not that *I'd* anything to snap out of. I wasn't the type to have psychological hang-ups, not me. Good for a laugh I'd always been, and good for a laugh I'd still be, but I told myself that the smiling face I presented to the world was merely a mockery of the deep and spiritual trauma through which I was passing.

I wanted . . . oh, I didn't know what I wanted. Perhaps the religious faith I'd known as a child and as an impressionable adolescent. I thought back to the days when, as a Methodist, I'd gone to Chapel Sunday morning and evening, sitting in a hard-backed pew, dressed in the coat kept specially for weekends, and listening, really listening to the sermon.

In the afternoon there would be Sunday School, and the Superintendent would talk to us about his love of God. Jesus had seemed to be a very real person to me then. We weren't clever enough to be cynical then.

Was that why we had such a happy acceptance?

Now I knew I didn't want the trappings of religion – the Churchianity as a friend called it – but the Christianity I'd known as a child. But now I was a grown woman, and my mind was cluttered with the whys and wherefores, and miracles didn't happen, not in this day and age, one only needed to pick up a newspaper to know that.

Then one day as I sat in front of my typewriter in my little room, trying to summon up the urge to lift the cover off it, the telephone rang.

Before I went into hospital I'd completed a novel, my first attempt at an adult full-length work, in spite of the dozens of serials and hundreds of short stories I'd written.

'Yes? Speaking,' I said.

And the voice at the other end was the publishing firm to which I'd sent my novel, and they liked it and wanted to buy it. . . .

I sat there for a long time after I'd replaced the receiver, then I rang the girls and told them, and they said they weren't surprised, not in the least.

Marilyn said it wouldn't be long before I was chatting up Michael Parkinson on his television show, and Kate said she just hoped I wouldn't sob and show them all up when they came through the curtains hand in hand with the grandchildren as Eamonn Andrews read out riveting little anecdotes about my life.

I had made Frank's favourite dish that evening, a cheese and bacon casserole, and we washed it down with a celebratory bottle of red wine. I told him the plots of my next three novels, and denied flatly that I'd said I wouldn't write again.

'Your voice sounds more like itself again,' a friend told me when I telephoned her the next evening.

'Anyone would think I'd been going around depressed or something,' I told Frank.

He grinned at me: 'It was the anaesthetic working itself gradually out through your pores after blocking up

152

your whole system, love,' he said.

So once again it no longer mattered that I was a prisoner in my own house. I was back in business again, and short stories winged their way to my editors. I still had arthritis, but the agonizing pain in my knee had gone.

I worked conscientiously at the exercises, sitting on the bed, pressing the back of my knee down hard, then relaxing with the radio going full strength, until eventually the slight 'lag' at the back of my leg had almost gone, and I was able to lie comfortably in bed with my leg stretched out flat again.

The newly-founded Arthritic and Rheumatism Club at the hospital held its monthly meetings, and I made new friends and overcame my reluctance at being one of a group sharing the same symptoms. I saw the pleasure it brought to men and women who were more crippled than I was, and wished every hospital in the country ran a similar scheme.

I was managing to get around the house without the aid of a stick, climbing the stairs helped by the extra-rail, taking a comfortable shower each morning seated on a special board placed across the bath, and attending the hospital for my weekly gold injection.

Every day I tried to walk a little further down the avenue, got to know a few more cats, and wrote and wrote and wrote.

A magazine telephoned one day and said they were sending a photographer round to take pictures to illustrate a two-part serial they were planning.

'As it's a family story, we would like the grandchildren there if possible,' they said, so I alerted the girls, and at the appointed time they all arrived.

Alison and Kathryn carried suitcases, and ran upstairs to change into their 'longs' for the first group of pictures. Their straight brown hair hung clean and shining, and Marilyn told me that they had been practising suitable expressions in front of the mirror at home for days.

Fortunately the photographer had children of his own, and was soon absorbed into the hurly-burly of a large family atmosphere, drinking coffee in the kitchen, and exuding endless patience with us all.

Jamie, aged four, went to lie down behind the sofa, and flatly refused to emerge.

'Boys don't like having their photographs taken,' he informed us from his prone position, just as Alison and Kathryn reappeared to take their places by my chair, gazing soulfully into the camera.

Lucy, their young sister, aged two, climbed on to my knee and kissed me.

The photographer thought that was great. 'Do that again, Lucy.' She obliged, making quite sure this time that her profile was turned towards the camera.

'Sit on Grandpa's knee,' said the photographer to Daniel of the bubbly curls and angelic smile, thus ensuring that a rather reluctant Frank would be in at least one of the photographs.

'Come and stand by Nannie,' said Kate to Jamie, 'There's a good boy.'

'I'll stand by her if I can look through the window,' said Jamie, and so there we were, the girls posing madly, Frank obviously wondering what he'd let himself in for, and Jamie, with his back to the camera, staring stolidly through the window.

'Say cheese,' said someone, and we all laughed, including Jamie, who forgot himself so far as to turn round just for a moment.

There was to be another set of pictures out in the garden, so Alison and Kathryn rushed upstairs again to change into what they considered more suitable, and Jamie went missing.

We found him sitting on the floor in my little study, busily drawing an exact replica of my operation scar on his knee with red pencil. It was a beauty, complete with stitch marks, and we praised his artistry so much that he allowed himself to be led outside, but warned us that he was going to keep his eyes closed.

The house and garden were full to overflowing with children, willing Mums, and none too willing Dads, and as we sat down to a cold lunch I looked round the crowded table and knew I was back in circulation once again.

Somehow, after thirty years, I knew I was finally coming to terms with the fact that I had arthritis, and I didn't need to pretend any more, not even to myself. Now I knew the enemy as I'd never known it before. I wasn't going to wear myself out pretending that I was a normal healthy woman, I was going to *accept* my disabilities and the inevitable slowing down of my lifestyle.

The hour after lunch lying on my bed would no longer be a habit I was ashamed of. If a friend telephoned and I was a long time answering, I wouldn't lie and say I'd been in the garden, but admit that I'd been resting.

I would admit that there were days when I couldn't get to my meetings, even with the help of a hired car, and without in the least giving in to my complaint, I would arrange my life to accommodate it.

Yes, gone were my days of wine and roses, perhaps for ever, but what was left was sweet, and infinitely worth while. I still counted my blessings, but now they were more simplified as I gave up striving for goals I couldn't reach.

I realized that there would, in all probability, be more operations ahead, because until a cure for arthritis is found, nothing but surgery can help joints that have been destroyed. And I am one of the lucky ones.

I have the love of my family and friends, plus the added bonus of an all-absorbing hobby. *I* can fight depression. I have to, for the sake of those I love, but for others, I realize, the way is doubly hard.

There are the men and women, severely crippled, struggling to live alone and retain their independence. I remember in particular the bright-eyed little widow in hospital who had a hip and both knees operated on, and still kept her Cockney sense of humour.

She told me how each morning she sat on the side of her bed, willing herself to make the supreme effort of getting a cup of tea. Completely alone and housebound, and yet still able to see the funny side of life. With both legs bandaged she was talking about the cruise she would go on when she could walk again.

She and her like are the courageous ones, not I.

So still I call on my mental Pollyanna, and still manage to live my life, if not to the full, in a privately satisfactory way. For example, one evening, not so long ago, we went out to dine at a rather trendy roadhouse.

I had taken an extravagant taxi to the hairdressers, and dressed with difficulty, but with care, my leg scar hidden beneath a long black skirt.

The head waiter relieved me of my stick, looping it reverently over the back of my chair, as carefully I avoided Frank's wink.

There was a four-piece band, and a postage-stamp sized floor, and in between the buttered shrimps and the fillet steak, the band started playing our tune.

A singer with a sob in his throat started to sing 'You made me love you', and it was a sentimental moment, it was corny, but Frank laid down his napkin and held out his hand.

'They're playing our tune. Shall we dance, love?' he said.

We were twenty years older, and maybe more, than the majority of the other couples on that tiny floor, and I could do no more than sway in time to the music, leaning heavily on him.

'You made me love you,' sang the leader of the band.

'And I didn't want to do it,' sang Frank with great feeling into my right ear.

And as we moved slowly, oh so slowly, I felt tears prick behind my eyelids, tears I'd sworn once I couldn't shed. Then, as the music changed tempo, we shuffled into a slow and laborious waltz, without the slightest regard for the clear and undisputed fact that it happened to be a rollicking rumba. . . .

# 15

It would be lovely if I could say that the wave of optimism and euphoria wafted us into membership of an old time dancing team, but as all arthritics know, the complaint can go into a period of remission.

This means that they, especially dunderheads like me, come to believe their symptoms have vanished, never to return. Alas, mine came back with a vengeance.

However, compensations there were a-plenty. To my amazement, my very first novel, *the Guilty Party*, was short-listed for the Romantic Novelist's Award, and I went all the way by taxi to the Park Lane hotel for the annual dinner, and saw my name printed on the menu.

I didn't win the award, but oh, the private joy of being short-listed! It made up for all the long lonely hours closeted in my little upstairs room. And it isn't true, as a famous columnist once stated, that romantic novelists all wear Fair-Isle berets and corduroy slacks. The ladies were dressed to kill in flowing gowns, and they were friendly, and yes, *loving*. I felt proud to be counted as one of them.

But insecure as ever, not knowing to which "genre" I rightly belonged, I wrote a murder story called *Footsteps in the Park*. I set it in the Lancashire of the thirties during the period of the Depression, a time of great hardship for the unemployed.

I discovered whilst writing this book that climbing the stairs to my little den was taking the edge off my creative urge. I would make endless excuses *not* to go to my typewriter, and it took a long time for the truth to dawn.

I wasn't reluctant to write; what I was reluctant to do was go up and down those flamin' stairs!

So, once again, Frank and I sat down and tried to work out a solution.

What we needed, we decided, was a bungalow within a stone's throw of the shops. Simple!

For the next two years we searched, only to discover that bungalows, surely needed most by elderly and disabled people, seem to be built in long winding avenues, as far from the shops as possible. Over and again we found what we wanted, only to realize that I would have been marooned, thus adding to my burden of guilt whenever I used a taxi.

We had almost given up when one morning, waiting to be picked up from the hairdresser's by the nice taxi man from the station forecourt, I glanced in the estate agent's window.

There was a bungalow advertized in a village a few miles away. The blurb made it sound as if the shops were indeed a mere hop, skip and jump away, which would have been good for a laugh even if I could hop, skip or jump, but when I told Frank he made an immediate appointment to view.

And the bungalow was white, neat and pretty, very close to a church, with the shops literally around the corner. It was called, much to my amusement, The Studio.

A great believer in signs from above, I whispered to Frank:

'Whoever lived here before must have been of artistic inclination.' And even without the Fair-Isle beret, surely that was me?

Hardly able to believe our luck, we followed the agent into the empty house. And there it was. An enormous sitting-room with five windows, long bookshelves already built in, a small kitchen with a dining-room, all the usual mod. cons, and at the front, overlooking the garden, a room which had once been a garage, designed exactly to take my desk, typewriter and overflow of books.

'It was waiting for us,' I told the bemused agent, a polite young man with a droopy moustache. 'All this time here it was, quietly waiting. Oh, can't you sense the atmosphere? It's like soft music playing.'

The moustache twitched slightly. 'Well, actually madam, I believe the first family to live here was musical. He was an organist, and the daughter was a concert pianist.'

'I knew it!' I cried, clasping my ugly hands together in ecstasy, while Frank tried to look not too ashamed of me.

So in the long hot summer of '76, we moved in. Both Marilyn and Kate were expecting babies, and in between their visits I was starting another novel, *Ring-a-Roses*. I was seeing myself this time as an historical novelist, finding the story fairly easy to write on two counts. The first was that history had always been my favourite subject at school, especially the Stuart period. The second was that sitting typing in a heat so intense, with my lard-white legs and arms for once bared to the air, I *identified*.

The summer of 1665 had been equally hot, and adding to the distress of the Londoners was the stench and rotted filth of a plague-ridden city. My characters were sweating, and so was I. Arthritis doesn't like hot humid weather, and by golly I was going to make my characters suffer even more!

I was typing damply one sweltering hot day when the telephone rang.

After I put the receiver down I tried to get back into the narrow streets of seventeenth-century London, but it was no good. My hero had just found a bubo beneath his left arm-pit, a sure sign of plague, and I didn't care.

As any professional writer knows, that is the time to call a halt, as not to care deeply about one's characters is fatal. I switched off my typewriter and went into the sitting-room, where two jolly men clad in white overalls were painting the walls and ceiling a brilliant white.

'All right, love?' The smaller decorator put down his brush to stare at me.

I said I didn't know.

'We heard the telephone ring. It's not bad news, is it?' He shifted a cigarette to the other side of his mouth, looking at me kindly.

For the week the two men had been working in the bungalow I had not had to supply them with a single cup of tea or coffee. On the first day they had told me it was their wont to bring their own refreshment with them. All I had to provide was the glasses – tumbler-size. As their refreshment consisted of gin and tonic drunk through smouldering cigarettes, they were the merriest decorators I have ever come across. At four o'clock in the afternoon their paint-splashed faces were glowing with bonhomie.

'My daughter has just phoned to say the clinic has told her the baby is a week overdue. Her *babies*,' I amended. 'She already has three little girls, and now she's going to have twins!'

My transition from professional writer to worried Lancashire mum was immediate and complete.

A large gin, splashed with a small tonic, was pressed into my hands, and before I could explain that I never drank gin, that even two small sherries rendered me paralytic, I was urged to drink it down.

'I told her,' I said, the gin bringing my sentimental streak to the surface already, "that God only sends twins to parents who can cope. And Marilyn and Bryan will cope. They have enough love for at least twenty children. Their house is always full of other people's children as well as their own.'

'Well, then,' said my jolly decorator, refilling my glass, and whipping the dust-sheet off a chair so that I could sit down.

So two days later Sarah and Emily arrived, as identical as peas in a pod, with round chubby faces and star-fish hands.

'Five girls,' my son-in-law said. 'And even the dog a bitch!'

By the end of the year *Ring-a-Roses* was finished. As most of the characters had died, it came to a natural end anyway. As I parcelled it up to send to my agent the telephone rang.

Kate had just given birth to her third son, a sturdy lad they called Tom.

When Mike ran me over to minister, I found Kate, just two days afterwards, stuffing washing in her machine, her elfin face a mask of determined exhaustion.

'Go and sit down, Mummy,' she told me. 'You look awful!'

Eight grandchildren . . . it was a lovely if sobering thought, and I wished I lived just around the corner so I could help out more. But even as I wished this I was gratefully acknowledging a truth.

With a mother suffering from arthritis for all their young lives, a mother who disappeared into hospital on twelve occasions, mostly for long periods, the two girls had grown up fiercely independent, more than able to survive. They are both far better cooks than I, who tends to drop things and make do with wrong ingredients to save walking to the shops.

So in that respect, the ill wind that gave me arthritis at the age of twenty-five blew total self-reliance their way. Not a bad thing at all.

Although my "new" knee was still working beautifully, my right one was becoming more swollen and painful, and my hands steadily more deformed. I wore long plaster splints at night, and working splints during the day to hold up my wrists, but mostly when I went out anywhere posh, I bandaged them tightly with crepe bandages which didn't show beneath long sleeves. I was old enough to admit even to myself now that I wasn't being brave, just vain.

Early in the new year I went to lunch with a different editor, a pretty, quiet girl whom I took to immediately.

Downing two glasses of wine too quickly, I was ready to bare my soul. Over the main course I told her a little about my own beginnings. About my mother dying in the infirmary giving birth to me; about the Sister who placed me as a tiny newborn baby in a soldier's bed for warmth; and about my lovely grandma who always called me her L'al lass. Herself over sixty, she had taken me from the infirmary, walking five miles through the streets with me wrapped in a shawl.

'She had brought up eleven children of her own, sending them all to work as weavers in the nearby cotton mill,' I confided dramatically over my glass of dry white wine. 'We were poor but honest, very respectable, strict church goers. My grandma was so puritanical that if any of her married daughters dared to sit with their feet apart, she would waft her hand to nudge them into closing their knees. There was always the smell of ox-tail stew simmering in the black fire-oven, and we washed in relays at the stone slop-stone in the living room. Only hands and face of course. The ruder parts were washed in a basin in the privacy of a bedroom.'

My editor was listening with a rapt expression on her face. She leaned forward. 'Have you ever written about that early environment, Marie?'

I shook my head. 'Never. Though I can't think why not. I published hundreds of short stories and never once touched on it.' I took a sip of wine. 'Strange.'

'Then I suggest you begin right now. You can super-impose fiction on the background you obviously know so well and remember with affection. Wouldn't you like to try?'

I nodded, ideas already walking round in my mind like unformed ghosts. I sent an outline to Mary, my agent, and immediately she gave me the encouragement that from the depths of her kindly wisdom she understands I need so much.

So *Maggie Craig* came to be written.

After three or four false starts – it isn't easy writing so

near to the bone – I set the book back in time. My grandma was a Cumberland woman, moving to the Lancashire cotton town on her marriage. I am lucky to have a retentive memory, almost total recall, so I was able to describe in detail the terraced house I remembered so vividly.

My mother had had a tragic life, even before losing it giving me birth. Her first husband was killed in France, going off after only two days of marriage together. My father I saw only a few times during my early childhood, but he had served in France, too, so the passages about Joe in *Maggie Craig* were written with extra feeling. The book was not in any way autobiographical, although I couldn't resist putting in the piece about the baby in the soldier's bed.

I was pointed out to the same soldier when I was about twelve years old. He was by then over his war wounds and was driving an ice-cream cart, and I remember blushing bright red at the inference that we had once shared the same bed.

So absorbed was I in writing about my own roots, it was as though I had never been away. I could still feel the horsehair sofa pricking my bare legs, still see the fire in the black-leaded grate, and the sharp tug on my scalp as my grandma wound my long hair into curling rags every night.

I was wallowing in memories, but in spite of my absorption my hands and arms were becoming less and less able to function. I had to resort to all kinds of gadgets to help me dress and shower.

But I hadn't time to *dwell*, thus proving what the medical profession has always believed. Arthritis can be greatly helped if the patient has an absorbing interest to lift the mind beyond the pain.

It was an easy step to my next novel, *A Leaf in the Wind*. Again using the background I remember so well, but setting the story back in time, I recalled a girl I once knew who had worked in a pet shop. Frank drove me over to a shop about four miles away, and there I struck lucky.

The owner, a tall man, twinkled down at me through his spectacles.

'My father owned a pet shop like this at the turn of the century, but then they were called cat meat shops. The cat meat was horse and sold mainly for dogs.' He grinned and launched into a description of the shop in those far-off days.

So, Jenny of the cat meat shop was born.

I was then attending, as I still am, a rheumatology clinic for my gold injections, each one of which has to be carefully monitored by blood tests and body weight. When surgery was considered for my hands it was agreed that I would continue for as long as possible with the splints. And anyway, I hadn't *time* to go back into hospital!

It was time, my editor told me, that I wrote a contemporary novel, and here I hadn't far to look for my heroine. Walking round our churchyard after morning service, I saw an ancient tombstone with the name EMMA SPARROW carved out in the weathered stone.

There she was, small, brown-haired and vulnerable, quick to react, weighed down at first by overwhelming odds. Now to find her an occupation? Lying in bed, I pondered.

A long time ago, waiting for the results of the Civil Service examinations to come out, I took a job in a clothing factory. I worked in a glass-fronted office, with a view of rows of benches manned by women machinists making raincoats. That was it!

But to bring my memories slap up to date I got out the Yellow Pages and rang around the local factories. To my delight a pleasant voice invited me to go and look around her factory which was just this side of Watford.

So off we went, and while Frank chatted up the supervisor – she was very dishy – I wandered about asking questions and imbibing the atmosphere. They were making high quality clothes, and as I listened and observed, Delta Dresses, the firm in my book came into focus.

Now all I had to do was write the book!

The twins and Tom were growing into non-stop chatterers, and on their weekly visits the cover went on my typewriter and I reverted to my other rôle, that of besotted grandma. So it wasn't much of a step to my next novel, *The Gemini Girls* – a story about identical twins, what else? The hero I called Tom, naturally!

My lovely grandma died when I was seven, in circumstances I haven't been able to write about as yet, and I went to live with my aunt and uncle in a house like the one I had described in *Maggie Craig*.

Uncle was a compositor on the local paper, an idealistic socialist of the old school, later to become a magistrate. Although I was much too young to remember the General Strike of 1926, I recollected now his description of it, and the effect it had on the working classes in the north of England. So with my mind walking round this period I wrote my synopsis. Once again fiction superimposed on fact.

It was about this time that Marilyn and family moved to Washington for four years, and although I was desolate at seeing them go, I was happy for them. Kate would miss them, too, as both families had spent holidays together, and Tom and the twins, being much of an age, were great friends.

I was thinking now around the idea of a novel set in the last war. Frank had flown on operations in the RAF, and promised to help with the technical details. So far so good. I tried to "see" my heroine. She would be a typical Lancashire lass, but she would be almost stone-deaf! This because, in spite of an operation, my own hearing leaves much to be desired. I cannot hear without a hearing-aid hidden underneath my hair, so I decided I would work out my frustrations on Sally in the next book.

During this time I was attending the hospital three times a week for hydrotherapy to try to straighten my right arm. I imagined myself swimming around in a sea-green pool, using my own peculiar brand of breast stroke. This consists of keeping my head up, well clear of the water, so not a strand of hair gets wet. I could even swim in my spectacles and not have them splashed!

But alas, the 'pool' was so small that I could have covered a length with two strokes. The water was very hot and my elbow was gently exercised beneath the surface, giving the arm a mobility I hadn't dreamed was possible. I was humbled by the dedication of the young physiotherapist standing with her patients in the steaming water for long hours, carefully moving their limbs up and down.

Working on the principle that travelling abroad is simpler for me than trudging round the supermarket, we flew the Atlantic to stay with Marilyn and family for two blissful weeks. The house was warm; *American* warm. The weather was the same, and I was wrapped around with affection, even by Marilyn and Bryan's American friends who treated us like life-long buddies.

Washington is a beautiful city with white buildings etched against a blue sky, so I feel sure that in my next novel one of my characters at least will find their way there during the story.

Since the first hardback edition of *One Step at a Time* was published I have received hundreds of letters on the subject of arthritis, the theme of almost every one of which has been loneliness. Pain can be a very lonely thing when borne alone.

The writers of these letters are the brave ones, not me. My own defence is not courage, but a loathing for sympathy. To illustrate my cowardly streak I need only mention when Frank nudged me on our recent flight in a jumbo-jet.

'If you look down you can see that we are flying over

Manhattan,' he enthused. 'Look! There's the Statue of Liberty.'

'No, thank you,' I said.

'Why on earth not?'

'Because I am on a bus,' I told him firmly.

I repeat, I am one of the lucky ones. My wrists may need to be supported all the time now, but I am still able to type my own rough drafts after a fashion. Bunty, my typist, herself a Lancashire woman, transforms my slip-shod typing into perfect copies, understanding the northern phraseology without the need for constant tele-phone calls for explanation. If my fingers have strayed on to the wrong keys she ignores the many alterations and turns out over a hundred thousand words without a single typing error.

So once again I thank God that finding out I had a certain flair for words at the age of forty proved to be my own small miracle.

Without this, and the support of my large and loving family; without the kindness and help I have always been shown by the doctors and nurses in various hospitals, I often wonder what sort of a woman I might have become?

Without my beloved typewriter and the creative out-let which came to me so unexpectedly, I might have had another tale to tell.

And without a tale to tell . . . ah, that would be unthinkable.

So it's on to the next book.

My own personal rather nauseating Pollyanna has triumphed once again!

*On the following pages are some of Marie Joseph's latest best-selling titles, also published by Arrow.*

# MAGGIE CRAIG

## Marie Joseph

*From the natural successor to Catherine Cookson*

At the turn of the century, the north of England was a hard, bleak world. A world where the only things in plenty were work and poverty – where joy and love were words in someone else's book. A world where men were resigned and women oppressed. It was here that Maggie Craig was born.

Strong-willed and spirited, as rebellious as she was beautiful, Maggie Craig flew in the face of the harshness of her life – and found a man she truly loved. But that passion was to cost her dearly all her life . . .

£1.50

# A LEAF IN THE WIND

## Marie Joseph

She was hardship's child – born to struggle and to serve.

He was fortune's favourite – born to flourish and be served.

They lived worlds apart. Jenny was the girl from the cat-meat shop, born into squalor and defeat. Paul Tunstall was a soldier and a gentleman, arrogant and charming, with his silver-light eyes and boyish smile. And yet from the moment they met there was a spark between them – and their separate lives of pain and loneliness seemed to beckon to each other.

But should she succumb to that plea in his eyes, to that longing in herself? Should she cross the line of class, the boundaries of propriety? Dare Jenny risk all to lose herself to love?

£1.50

# FOR THE LOVE OF ANN

## James Copeland

'The doctor cleared his throat and spoke very quietly. "I am so very sorry to have to tell you this, but I'm afraid that our tests show that it is extremely unlikely that your daughter will ever be educated, or for that matter, that she will ever be able to recognise you as her parents".'

That was 1958, and Ann Hodges was six years and eight months old. Today that same girl is in her twenties. Full of charm. Devoted to her parents and her brothers and excitedly taking in the world and its challenges.

Between those two dates lies a remarkable story. A love story born out of hopelessness and ignorance and nurtured in years of tears and joy . . . *all for the love of Ann.*

75p

# HEARTSOUNDS

## Martha Weinman Lear

On 10 August 1973, Dr Harold Lear, 52, suffered a major coronary. *Heartsounds* is the story of the years that followed. It is an account of medical drama and medical failure; of individual fear, courage and vulnerability; of a couple forced for the first time to question their life; of a doctor who, as a patient, finds himself doubting the assumptions on which his profession had been based.

But even more, it is a love story – the story of two people made to look deeply and honestly at themselves and their marriage by a crisis that daily threatens tragedy.

'An awesome and gripping book . . . absorbing, wild, funny, tender, enraging and absolutely remarkable' *New York Book Review*

'A testament to the power of human love and the will to live' *Publishers Weekly*

'Engrossing, touching and frightening' *Washington Post*

£1.75

# BESTSELLERS FROM ARROW

All these books are available from your bookshop or news-agent or you can order them direct. Just tick the titles you want and complete the form below.

| | | |
|---|---|---|
| PROMISES | Charlotte Vale Allen | £1.95 |
| THE AFTER DINNER GAME | Malcolm Bradbury | £1.75 |
| THE KGB DIRECTIVE | Richard Cox | £1.75 |
| MCENROE | Tania Cross | £1.50 |
| GOD BLESS THE BORDERS! | Lavinia Derwent | £1.25 |
| WELLIES FROM THE QUEEN | Colin Douglas | £1.50 |
| A DISTANT SUNSET | Virginia Ironside | £1.50 |
| ONE STEP AT A TIME | Marie Joseph | £1.50 |
| PAINTED BIRD | Jerzy Kosinski | £1.60 |
| SCANDALS | Barney Leason | £1.95 |
| THE CHAMDO RAID | John Miller | £1.60 |
| PIN | Andrew Neiderman | £1.50 |
| WHITENIGHTS, RED DAWN | Frederick Nolan | £1.95 |
| TORPEDO RUN | Douglas Reeman | £1.50 |
| WOLF TO THE SLAUGHTER | Ruth Rendell | £1.50 |
| THE EXPERIMENT | Richard Setlowe | £1.75 |
| SONGS FROM THE STARS | Norman Spinrad | £1.75 |
| MORE TALES FROM A LONG ROOM | Peter Tinniswood | £1.50 |
| THE FACTS OF RAPE | Barbara Toner | £1.75 |
| THE CLAW OF THE CONCILIATOR | Gene Wolfe | £1.60 |

Postage _____

Total _____

---

**ARROW BOOKS, BOOKSERVICE BY POST, PO BOX 29, DOUGLAS, ISLE OF MAN, BRITISH ISLES**

Please enclose a cheque or postal order made out to Arrow Books Limited for the amount due including 10p per book for postage and packing for orders within the UK and 12p for overseas orders.

*Please print clearly*

NAME ...............................................

ADDRESS ...........................................

..................................................

Whilst every effort is made to keep prices down and to keep popular books in print, Arrow Books cannot guarantee that prices will be the same as those advertised here or that the books will be available.